What's Going on Down There?

What's Going on Down There?

Improve Your Pelvic Health

Dr. Sam Siddighi and Dr. Neil Baum
with Michelle Fitzpatrick

Book cover design by Eduardo Davad
Illustrator Gary Hallgren

Library of Congress Control Number: 2012912213
ISBN: Hardcover   978-1-4771-4023-9
                Softcover   978-1-4771-4022-2
                Ebook   978-1-4691-1099-8

printed in china by artful dragon press, a u.s. company

To order additional copies of this book, contact:
Xlibris Corporation
1-888-795-4274
www.Xlibris.com
Orders@Xlibris.com
113198

CONTENTS

Medical Disclaimer

Dedication

I dedicate this book to my wife, whose support has made my participation possible, and whose gift of my two children is the best I ever had. Of all that walk the earth, you three are the most precious to me. I also want to thank my patients for inspiring me to write this book.

Sam Siddighi

This book has been made possible by the hard work and dedication of my co-authors, my family, and my patients. Michelle Fitzpatrick and Dr. Sam Siddighi have worked diligently to translate medical jargon into information that is easy for all women to understand—and to put into practice. I would also like to thank my wife, Linda, and my three children who are my inspiration and my greatest source of pride. Finally, I would like to acknowledge my wonderful patients who have provided me with their stories about challenges that have occurred down there—their openness will help generations of women better understand how to address their concerns more quickly and comfortably.

Neil Baum

Foreword

This book is an awesome tool for all women. I really wish I had had this book right after my first child was born in 1998. I too am one of those women who lived in silence about what I realized was a real medical issue stress incontinence. At first I didn't talk about it with my husband or my sister, who has kids and is a nurse. However, one year was long enough for me before I went to the doctor and started asking questions. But many women wait 5 to 10 years before seeking help. This book provides much-needed answers to many women's health issues. As I near perimenopause, I find this book to be useful to me in my present life. It really is for women of varying ages, as we all go through things at different times and stages of our lives. I love how the authors provide information on different medicines, lists of questions to ask your doctor, and drawings that help with understanding it all—not to mention everything is in layman's terms. Thanks for putting this resource together to answer all our questions about "down there."

Bonnie Blair
Four-time Olympian with five Gold Medals
and one Bronze Medal, mother of two,
and former "down there" patient

"This extraordinarily informative book for women over 40 is precisely what its authors claim it to be: a confidence-boosting guidepost for women to use with their doctors that allows them to communicate effectively their wishes and thereby share actively in decisions about, and care for, their own pelvic health and related emotional needs. It is written in a direct, conversational tone but with all the details needed to fully educate a mature woman about her anatomy, her options, her risks, and her rights. All surgical procedures a woman might consider are described succinctly, with the pros and cons of each. Even labiaplasty is addressed so that women know when they might consider it and what to expect. It's all here, without omission of any important topic, covered with a no-nonsense, knowledgeable, and practical voice that is open and not judgmental. It is full of good preventive tips, too—such as how to lift to avoid straining muscles and inducing prolapse—and tackles the most delicate of topics with directness and accuracy—such as fecal incontinence and chronic constipation. PMS is taken seriously and given its own chapter, and the book concludes with a helpful, detailed checklist of what to expect for pre-and post-operative care surrounding surgery and a top 10 list of stress relievers. Given the fact that over a woman's lifetime, 11% are likely to undergo pelvic surgery for incontinence or prolapse and 29% will have repeat procedures, not to mention other pelvic health and sexual concerns, no woman over 40 should be without this book."

Nancy Muller, PhD, MBA
Executive Director
National Association For Continence
www.nafc.org

Introduction

If you are a woman between the ages of 40 and 90 and you have one or more of a dozen of issues that occur in a woman's pelvis, where do you turn for help? Online sources provide an abundance of information, but how do you know which are credible? How do you make sense of all the information you have found on the Internet? Oftentimes, bookstores and Amazon.com provide books written in very technical language, and the solutions they provide are often difficult to understand.

Why did we write this book? We have visited dozens of bookstores, read hundreds of books on the topics included in this book, and have not found a single book that provided practical, credible, and easy-to-understand concepts regarding women's pelvic health. We have had so many patients in our practice ask us questions about their pelvic health, and we felt there was a need for a book that provides answers for patients before they seek medical advice. Many women have only vague symptoms and have difficulty articulating their complaints to their physicians. Both of us have had patients who just complain about not being quite right "down there." We hope this book will educate, inform, and empower women to clearly articulate what is bothering them. So when the doctor asks what is wrong, they can respond with a concise and clear explanation, and be forthright, detailed, and specific about their issues.

We have taken hundreds of years of medical knowledge pertaining to women's health issues including the latest medical breakthroughs and have distilled it down to the most important and easy to understand for anyone who is reading this book. As of the writing of this book, there is no other book available that discusses all the topics detailed in this book and in such a way to make it easily understandable, practical, and useable for the lay, nonmedical woman.

We have written a book that covers the most common female medical conditions (i.e., menopause, vaginal prolapse, hysterectomy, accidental bowel leakage, premenstrual syndrome, pelvic pain, urinary incontinence, vaginal rejuvenation, stress, and others) that affect the nearly 65 million women in the United States above the age of 40. And this number is expected to almost double by 2020. We have deliberately excluded conditions such as sexually transmitted diseases, female infertility, pregnancy, and basic gynecologic issues as these conditions usually pertain to women younger than 40, and there are numerous credible sources of information about them. In addition, we do not discuss breast disease as this is beyond our areas of expertise, and there are many other books that have already illuminated this important topic.

This book is written by two expert physicians in the fields of gynecology and urology. We have 40-plus years of combined experience treating down there conditions. Our two areas of specialty in medicine are in a unique position to answer all the questions that women have regarding their pelvic tissues and female medical conditions. We both have academic appointments and are published authors in these topics. More importantly, we know firsthand the limited information available to our female patients, as well as their general lack of understanding and the challenges associated with asking the right questions of themselves and their healthcare providers.

We have combined our knowledge and passion by collaborating with two very talented individuals who have added another dimension to our book. Our collaborating writer, Michelle "Billie" Fitzpatrick, has done a tremendous job of organizing our writing and converting it into prose that is easy to read and really makes sense to women with no medical background. We are also fortunate to be able to work with Gary Hallgren, who is a genius medical illustrator, who, among other accolades, has created all the drawings for Dr. Roizen and Oz's popular *You Books*. The four of us have assembled a book that we feel will benefit all women, regardless of their age, their medical problems, and their medical background.

The problems that we discuss in this book are extremely common, and yet the majority of women know very little (if anything) about these conditions. Because of the thousands of patients that we have treated over the years, we have learned that these down there conditions are not discussed among friends, mothers, daughters, sisters, and grandmothers. In fact, our patients are often perplexed when we first tell them their diagnoses. We often hear comments such as, "I didn't know that was possible," or "I have never heard of that before," or "Why didn't my mother tell me this could happen?" We have both seen educated women from all walks of life who have a grapefruit-size fleshy protrusion from their vagina, and their best description of what is happening to them is, "Something is not right down there." We have also seen women that appear to be living normal lives, but unbeknownst to their family and friends are spending thousands of dollars on pads or diapers and dealing with their problems in secret. Why are they living this way? Why are they suffering in silence? We want to show you that it doesn't have to be that way. Help is available, and we are going to tell you how to find the source of your problem and even how to find a physician who can help you.

This book is intended to give you insight and knowledge about these very common conditions that you or a loved one may have. We want you to be aware that urinary incontinence *is not* a normal part of aging; sex *is* and can be enjoyable when you get older; and menopause *can* be the best time in your life. Thanks to the tremendous advancements doctors and scientists have made, most of the conditions we discuss are completely treatable.

We want to empower you so that you know when you should seek a second opinion. We have both had patients who, after mustering the courage to ask their doctor, were told that "not much can be done for that," or "that is what happens when you age." Some of our patients blatantly were given the wrong information. Women have been told that "it can't be fixed" or that the "treatments do not last." It is no wonder that by the time our patients see us, they have been suffering in silence with these down there conditions for at least five years. Hopefully, reading this book will prevent this from happening to you. By reading this book, you will become confident about your choice of doctor and treatment plan. Knowing about your condition will make you a more educated patient. When you do find the right doctor, you will become a better partner with your doctor and help him/her to make the best healthcare decision for you.

We don't want you to be embarrassed to talk to your friends, family, or doctor. It is okay to talk about the issues with the tissues down there. We hope that you will gather enough courage to join or even form your own book club to discuss the stories that were told in this book. To help you, we have included a list of discussion topics at the end of the book, if you are interested in participating in a book club.

If we have to recommend two books on female pelvic health, we suggest *What's Going on Down There?* and suggest you read it twice!

Chapter One

What's Going on Down There?
How to Understand Your Pelvic Health

Can you imagine a medical problem that affects every woman at some time in her life? If you answered breast disease, heart disease, arthritis, or depression, then you are wrong. The answer lies in the organs between a woman's navel and her knees. That's right, it's the organs in her pelvis: the uterus, the ovaries, the bladder, the vagina, and the rectum. Every woman at some time in her life will have a problem with one or more of these organs.

There are 156 million females in the United States and 65 million are over the age of 40; and every one of them has some issue or concern that affects the organs in the pelvis. Unfortunately, women often have to go to several doctors to try and find the answers to these problems, and sometimes they will suffer for years before a solution is found. Many women suffer in silence as they are uncomfortable discussing these problems with their significant others, their friends, and even with their doctors.

The two of us have nearly four decades of experience caring for women with problems in their pelvis. Both of us have encountered far too many women who come for a consultation after seeing 5 to 10 other physicians over many years and never receiving a diagnosis or effective treatment. Many women have been told that their pelvic pain, painful intercourse, or need to urinate 30 times a day was "in their heads" and that they were depressed and needed to see a psychiatrist or a mental health expert. The truth of the matter is that many of these women can be cured of their pelvic dysfunctions, nearly everyone can be helped, and the mental anguish and even the depression lifts when the problem in the pelvis is treated.

After years of seeing women in pain and their lives ruined by problems in the pelvis, we decided to write this book. We went to the Internet and typed in *"pelvic dysfunction"* and came up with over nine million hits, over two million for the topic of urinary incontinence, one million for pelvic organ prolapse, and half a million for painful intercourse. Unfortunately, most of the information we found on the Internet was inaccurate and not written by credible sources. And when we did find accurate information, there was too much detail, and it was written in medical jargon, making it almost impossible for someone who is not in the medical profession to understand it. This was a problem! As specialists in women's pelvic health, we realized there was a dire need for a complete, reliable, and relatable guide that helped women understand what was going on in their bodies—especially with the organs and tissues down there. We came to the conclusion that we had to write this guide to help the millions of women suffering from incontinence, constipation, painful bladder syndrome, female sexual dysfunction, prolapse, and a host of health issues that arise as women age, before, during, and after menopause.

This book is not intended as a self-help book but a guideline for women to use with their physician. This book is not intended so that women can diagnose and treat these pelvic problems. This book is written so that women will be enlightened about pelvic disorders and will have a greater understanding of these problems. As a result, women will know what kind of doctor they should see, what questions they should ask, and what results they may achieve.

We know from our combined 40 years in medical practice that women who are educated about their condition are much more confident and able to communicate better with their doctor. A doctor always appreciates if a patient has taken the time to become knowledgeable about her condition. It clearly demonstrates that the patient is becoming a partner in the relationship with the physician, and that by working together, they can function as a team to find the best possible solution to the problem.

We have worked with thousands of patients who present with these problems of their pelvic organs and have seen the quality of their lives improve significantly. Most of these problems are not killers or causes of death but are issues that "steal the lives" of women who suffer from pelvic dysfunctions.

We have seen women with urinary incontinence (involuntary loss of urine discussed in Chapter Two) who wear diapers or who spend a majority of their day looking for restrooms or sitting on a toilet. These are women who have become reclusive and are too embarrassed to socialize because of their incontinence and are embarrassed when they go to the drugstore and buy a box of Depend™ in order to avoid soiling their clothing. When these women are cured of their incontinence, their lives are turned around. They arrive with a smile on their face, they are interested in socializing once again, and they are delighted not to have to depend on Depend™!

We have seen women who have a lifelong history of painful intercourse (dyspareunia discussed in Chapter Eight). It is common for women with painful intercourse to avoid sexual intimacy with their partner. As a result, the couple has an unhappy relationship, which can lead to dissolution of the relationship, depression, and obstacles to effective and meaningful communication. Most women with dyspareunia can be helped and can put sexual intimacy back into their relationships.

Young girls often have difficulty making the transition from adolescence to puberty. This is a time when the female hormones, estrogen and progesterone, kick in, and young girls are becoming physiologically mature women (Chapter Six). There is also another important transition from childbearing to menopause. This too is a time of hormonal disarray. In Chapter Nine, we will discuss menopause and how women can move smoothly through it without the attendant symptoms such as hot flashes, irritability, and mood swings.

Indeed, the title of this book, *What's Going on Down There?*, is not merely a euphemism but a true reflection of the reality that most women experience when discussing pelvic organ problems with their doctors. Both of us (Dr. Siddighi and Dr. Baum) have seen women who cannot describe their complaints when they involve conditions affecting their pelvic organs. If they had a pain in their ankle or a headache, they could pinpoint the exact place where the discomfort exists, tell the doctor how long the pain has been there, and describe what circumstances aggravate and relieve the discomfort. However, they could have a grapefruit-sized mass protruding from their vagina and tell the doctor, "I don't feel quite right down there!" Women have difficulty describing the vague symptoms associated with pelvic malfunction. It is our purpose that those who read this book will have the information that they need to be able to better communicate the symptoms in the pelvis with their physicians. It is our intention that women will never have to use the expression *down there* again when they seek medical help for issues of the tissues in the pelvis!

Your Anatomy

This book addresses the down there of a woman's body, essentially all the organs and tissues of the pelvis. So although we will talk about other health issues, including gastrointestinal, circulatory, nervous, and other systems of the body, our main focus and concern are problems related to all that involves the urinary and reproductive systems.

To get started, we think it might be helpful to offer you a bit of a roadmap of where everything is located down there. You'd be surprised how many women are not exactly sure of their own anatomy.

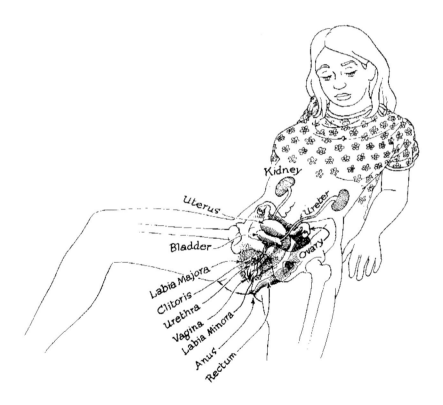

Vagina—the Passageway

The vagina is like a passageway between two places. The vagina is a muscular tube that forms a part of the female sex organs and which connects the neck of the uterus (called the cervix) with the external genitals. The vagina, which is approximately two and one-half to four inches long, has muscular walls, which are supplied with numerous blood vessels. These walls become erect when a woman is aroused as extra blood is pumped into these vessels. During arousal, fluid also enters through these vessels into the vagina giving the sensation of wetness. The vagina has three functions: as a receptacle for the penis during intercourse, as an outlet for blood during menstruation, and as a passageway for the baby to pass through at birth.

Vulva—the Package

The vulva is made up of several female organs, which are external. These include a small rounded pad of fat, which protects the pubic bone. Reaching down almost to the anus are two folds of fatty tissue called the larger lips, or labia majora, to protect the inner genitals. Just inside are two smaller lips, or labia minora, which enclose the opening of the urethra (which comes down from the bladder) and the vagina. At the upper end are small projections called the prepuce, which protect the clitoris.

Labia—the Doorway

The labia are the doorways to your external genitals. The labia (singular, labium) minora are flattened lengthwise into folds located with the cleft between the labia majora. These folds are composed of connective tissue that is richly supplied with blood vessels, causing a pinkish appearance. In the back, near the anus, the labia minora merge with the labia majora; while in the front, they converge to form a hoodlike covering around the clitoris. The labia majora refers to the large or outer lips. The labia majora start at the thigh and extend inward, surrounding the rest of the vulva. The outer edges are hair covered, the inner edges are smooth. The skin of the outer lips is rich in blood vessels and darker than the skin of the thighs. During arousal, the labia majora swell and become even darker.

The Bladder—an Expanding and Contracting Balloon

The urinary bladder acts like a balloon-like storage container that holds liquid waste until it is possible to evacuate the waste material from the body, expanding and contracting with urine rather than air. The bladder is a muscular sac in the pelvis, just above and behind the pubic bone. When empty, the bladder is about the size and shape of a pear; however, when the bladder is full of urine, it can reach the size of a grapefruit. Most women have two kidneys that act as a filter to remove liquid wastes from the body. Urine is made in each kidney and travels down a tube called the ureter to the bladder. The bladder stores urine, allowing urination to be infrequent and voluntary. During urination, the bladder muscles contract, and sphincters (valves) around the urethra open and relax to allow urine to flow outside the body.

The Urethra—the Stem of the Balloon

The urethra is a tube that conveys urine from the urinary bladder to the outside of the body. Its wall is lined with mucous membranes and contains a relatively thick layer of smooth muscle tissue. It also contains numerous mucous glands called urethral glands, which secrete mucus into the urethral canal. In females the urethra is less than 2 inches long. It passes forward from the bladder, descends below the symphysis pubis, and empties between the labia minora. Its opening is located above the vaginal opening and about 1 inch below the clitoris.

The Cervix—a Tube Stopper

The lower one-third of the uterus is the tubular cervix, which extends downward into the upper portion of the vagina. The cervix surrounds the opening called the cervical os, through which the uterus communicates with the vagina. The cervix functions like a plug or a stopper on a bottle. The cervix allows the entrance of sperm to fertilize the egg and then allows the exit of the baby during vaginal birth. The cervix is the location where a Pap smear is taken. It is also the area that opens, or dilates, during childbirth.

Clitoris—the Pleasure Zone

The clitoris is a sensitive organ with numerous nerve endings that, like the penis, contains tissues that fill with blood when sexually aroused.

The area of the clitoris that you can see and feel is only the tip of the iceberg. It is like a tuning fork that resonates when stimulated at the right frequency. The clitoris looks like a wishbone and is actually a long structure that increases in size when stimulated to almost four inches in length. The stimulation of the clitoris accounts for a large part of the physical pleasure during sexual intimacy.

The Fallopian Tubes—Your Delivery Tubes

The Fallopian tubes lie in the pelvic portion of the abdominal cavity, and each tube reaches from an ovary to become the upper part of the uterus. This funnel-shaped tube is about three inches in length and enables transport of egg and sperm during fertilization. The larger end of the funnel is divided into feathery, fingerlike projections that lie close to the ovary. These beating projections, along with muscle contractions, force the ovum down the funnel's small end, which opens into the uterus. The Fallopian tubes are like hoses that rhythmically expand and contract, expanding and contracting to move a fertilized egg from the ovary to the uterus where the embryo will be nourished and grow to a fetus until the fetus is ready to enter the real world as a baby.

The Kidneys—the Body's Filters

The kidneys are the filters that remove wastes that are excreted in urine. The kidneys are very sophisticated sieves that allow blood to enter. The kidneys then select the products that are to be kept in circulation and allow the liquid waste products to become urine to be excreted or removed from the body. The kidneys are located about two inches above the body's midpoint just below and behind the liver in the upper abdomen and behind the lower ribs. They are the balancers of internal fluids; so if we overeat or overdrink one day and diet the next, or if we have an active day, the kidneys will compensate and see that these fluctuations in fluid, salt, and glucose are leveled out. The kidneys are like sophisticated thermostats, and if too much fluid is in the body, the kidneys will reduce the body's fluid volume by making more urine. On the other hand, if the body is dehydrated, the kidneys will function to save fluid by decreasing the urine output.

Ovaries—The Egg-cubator

The ovaries are a pair of oval or almond-shaped glands that lie on either side of the uterus and just below the opening to the fallopian tubes. In addition to producing eggs or ova, the ovaries produce the female sex hormones estrogen and progesterone. A baby girl is born with about 1-2 million of these cells; and at puberty, there are 400,000 ova. However, there are only 400 ova that have the potential to be fertilized, which closely corresponds to the 400 periods a woman will have over her lifetime.

The Uterus-Baby Factory

The uterus or womb is a hollow, muscular organ that lies in the pelvic cavity behind the bladder and in front of the bowel. The uterus usually tilts forward at a 90-degree angle to the vagina, although in about 20 percent of women, it tilts backward. The uterus is lined with tissues that change during the menstrual cycle. These tissues build under the influence of hormones from the ovary. When the hormones withdraw before the menstrual cycle, the blood supply is cut off, tissues are shed as waste, and the unfertilized eggs die and become absorbed by the body. During pregnancy, the uterus stretches from three to four inches in length to a size that will accommodate a growing baby.

The Rectum—Waste Container

The rectum is a short muscular tube that forms the lowest portion of the large intestine and connects it to the anus. Feces collects here until pressure on the rectal walls cause nerve impulses to pass to the brain, which then sends messages to the voluntary sphincter muscles in the anus to relax, permitting expulsion of the solid waste material.

A woman's genital area is made up of three openings: the vaginal opening, which leads to the vagina; an anus, which leads to the rectum (the end of the large intestine, or colon); and a urinary opening, which leads to the urethra, a short (about an inch and a half) thin tube leading to your bladder. (Men, in contrast, have only two openings—the urethra and anus.) The urinary opening permits urination; the anus allows bowel movements; and the vaginal opening enables menstruation, sex, and birth of a child.

Getting Started

One of the main takeaways from this book will not only be accurate information and insight into what is going on down there, but also how to find the best doctor or practitioner to help you with your problem. When you want to buy an SUV or a hardwood kitchen flooring, you can study *Consumer Reports* and make an educated decision about that purchase. What do you do when you want to have cosmetic surgery or LASIK eye surgery? Worse yet, what do you do when you need to have a more esoteric type of procedure such as pelvic organ prolapse surgery or stool incontinence surgery? What type of surgeon specializes in that type of surgery? How do you find the right surgeon? These questions may be difficult to answer, and finding such a surgeon can be a daunting task if you don't know where to look. Unlike European countries, where the names of all the surgeons who are qualified to perform the type of surgery that you need are listed in alphabetical order in a government-run registry, such directories don't exist in the United States.

Finding the Right Doctor for You

Talk to Your Primary Care Provider

Talking with your family physician, internal medicine doctor, physician assistant, or nurse practitioner is a good place to start. Not only do they know your medical history, they also will know the type of specialty that deals with the kind of problem that you may be experiencing. They may be aware through word of mouth and community reputation who are the reputable surgeons in your community. This being said, they are also more likely to refer you to colleagues or friends. This may be bad or good depending on the situation. To remedy this possible bias, you should ask to talk to patients who have had surgery by the surgeon whom your primary care provider has recommended. It would be even more helpful if you can obtain the name of a couple of patients from your primary care provider who have had the *same type of surgery* that you need by the recommended surgeon. Then you can decide for yourself what kind of care you will be receiving from that potential surgeon. You can also ask your potential surgeon for a couple of references. However, as is human nature, you will be more likely to receive names of patients who have had the best outcome, and thus, they may not be representative of the typical patient that your potential surgeon treats. Most doctors are comfortable with giving you a couple of names of patients who you can call as references. (The person being called will have already given her permission so there is no violation of patient privacy.) In our practices, we have several patients who have had elective procedures agree to take calls from patients. The interested patient is given only the patient's phone number and not her name. This method preserves the patient's confidentiality. However, it's just as if not more common for willing patients to exchange names and agree to meet in person to discuss the surgery in greater detail.

Ask Family and Friends

If you have any family or friends who themselves have undergone surgery by a surgeon, then that can be a good source of information regardless of whether it is negative or positive. For instance, if your mother had a prolapse surgery by surgeon Z but was dissatisfied with some or all aspects of her care by that surgeon, then you may want to avoid that surgeon. On the other hand, it is comforting to get a recommendation from a close friend who has had a positive experience with a surgeon. If your family or friend happens to work in the healthcare field (i.e., doctor, nurse, nurse practitioner, physician assistant, or hospital employee), then the advice they give you probably is even more reliable. The healthcare community is not as big as you may think. Your family or friend can ask around for you and help you figure out who you should go to.

Ask Your Health Insurance Company

Depending on your health insurance company, this may be a good source of information. Your insurance company will always try to direct you toward an in-network physician. Your insurance company will know based on your diagnosis which doctors within network treat your condition. If you decide to choose an out-of-network surgeon, then you may be responsible for a higher percentage of the expenses. However, sometimes this may be the best thing to do if the in-network physician is not the most qualified or you don't feel comfortable with him/her.

Do Internet Research

You can find a vast amount of information on the Internet. The hard part is to know which websites provide accurate and reliable information. When it comes to finding the right surgeon, the Internet can also be another source of information. However, we would recommend that you not make your decision of which surgeon to choose based solely on the ratings provided by these websites as they are not always entirely accurate. A couple of sites that provide good information are Avvo.com and Healthgrades.com.

Many doctors post their patients' testimonials on their websites. This is certainly a source of information. But again, we advise you not to base your entire decision on just these testimonials because they may be biased. Only the best outcomes are chosen and included on these websites.

You can also find names of surgeons in your area that perform the type of surgery that you require. For urogynecologic and pelvic floor conditions, you can go to the websites of the following societies: American Urogynecologic Society (www.augs.org), Society of Urodynamics and Female Urology (www.sufuorg.com), American Congress of Obstetricians and Gynecologists (www.acog.org), American Urologic Association (www.auanet.org).

You can also use the Internet to exclude potentially bad doctors. Go to the US Department of Health and Human Services website to search the National Practitioners Data Bank (www.npdb-hipdb.hrsa.gov). You can research whether your potential surgeon has had any malpractice judgements or adverse disciplinary actions. You can also find contact information pertaining to your state medical board, which can be a source of additional information about your potential surgeon (read near the end of the document for state board information: www.npdb-hipdb.hrsa.gov/resources/NPDBGuidebook.pdf#page=25).

If you had to choose an interior decorator to furnish your home, we are guessing that you would at least talk to a couple of qualified decorators before you chose one of them. Since surgery can be a scarier and more life-altering event than selecting furnishings for your home, you should exercise due diligence in finding your surgeon. Take the time and effort to find the right person. Once you have done your research and have come up with at least two or three names of potential surgeons by following the steps that we have discussed above, you are now ready to take the next step. We would recommend that you see and obtain the opinions of two reputable surgeons. Why? Because surgeons are not created equal, and there may be differences in training, experience, and skill. There may be more than one approach or surgical technique to solve a problem. You may have a better connection with one over another. Additionally, it is better to go to a surgeon who can offer you several ways to treat your condition, discuss the advantages and disadvantages of each, and then guide you to choose the one method that suits you best.

Talk to the Nurses and Anesthesiologists

In our opinion, the nurses and the anesthesiologists at the surgeon's hospital are the best source of information regarding a surgeon's performance. Since the hospital nurses are not employed by the doctor and see patients from many surgeons, they are more objective in their assessment of how good a surgeon really is. On the other hand, speaking to the nurses at the surgeon's clinic or office may not be as reliable, since the surgeon employs those nurses. When you go to the surgeon's hospital, ask the nursing director or charge nurse to speak to the operating room nurses, the anesthesiologist, and floor nurses who cover your potential surgeon's patients. When you talk to them, make sure to pay attention to their nonverbal cues since most people will not say negative things about a doctor. Ask them, "Would you have surgery by doctor X?" If they are overwhelmingly positive and say they have recommended or are going to send their family or friend to that surgeon, then that is the best type of recommendation you can hope for. On the other hand, if they don't directly answer your question, or they tell you that doctor X is such a nice man/woman, then beware. You should speak to more than one person so you can be sure you have a balanced opinion of your potential surgeon. If everyone you speak to has the same opinion of your potential surgeon, then chances are that they are true.

Qualifications

Female pelvic medicine and reconstructive surgeons, female urologists, urologists, gynecologists, urogynecologists, and colorectal surgeons treat the conditions discussed in this book (see Table 1).

Table 1. Type of specialists who treat pelvic floor problems

Conditions requiring surgery	Specialty of your surgeon	Discussed in detail in chapter XYZ
Pelvic organ prolapse	FPMRS, FU, UG, G, U	Chapter Three
Urinary incontinence	FPMRS, FU, U, UG, G	Chapter Two
Stool/fecal incontinence	CRS, FPMRS, UG	Chapter Seven
Complications of above surgeries such as voiding problems, closed/constricted vagina, genital fistula, scarring, adhesions, mesh erosion	FPMRS, CRS, FU, UG, U	Chapters Two, Three, Seven, and Eight
Hysterectomy	G, FPMRS, UG	Chapter Ten
Vaginal tightening or labial surgery for medical reasons	FPMRS, UG, G	Chapter Eleven
Vaginal rejuvenation and cosmetic labial surgery*	G, PS, FPMRS	Chapter Eleven

Sexual dysfunction and painful intercourse related to previous surgery	FPMRS, UG, G	Chapter Eight
Vulvodynia, decreased libido, sexual pain disorders not related to surgery	G, U, UG, FPMRS	Chapter Eight

* Vaginal rejuvenation is a controversial topic, and many surgeons from these specialties do not perform this type of surgery (please see Chapter Eleven).

CRS = colon and rectal surgeon
FPMRS = female pelvic medicine and reconstructive surgery
FU = female urology
G = gynecology
PS = plastic surgery
UG = urogynecology
U = urology

All these doctors have finished four years of medical school to obtain an MD, medical degree. All of them have also completed four to five years of residency training beyond medical school. In addition, some of these doctors have also completed training for one to three years beyond residency (called fellowship) in order to become super-specialized in management of pelvic disorders (see Table 1). Fellowship training programs in female pelvic medicine and reconstructive surgery (FPMRS) and female urology (FU) are still in their early stages. There are not many surgeons with training in FPMRS. Thus, urogynecologists, experienced urologists, and gynecologists probably perform the vast majority of pelvic floor surgeries in your community.

Having a membership in the American Congress of Obstetricians and Gynecologists, the American College of Surgeons, and American Urologic Association can also be an indicator of achieving a level of ethical standards. If a surgeon has FACOG or FACS after his/her last name, this means the surgeon is a Fellow of the American Congress of Obstetricians and Gynecologists or Surgery, respectively. Do not confuse the term fellow in FACOG/FACS with doing fellowship training because they are not the same thing (as explained in the previous paragraph). You can either ask your potential surgeon about his/her membership or look at the initials after his/her name. Not having initials after their name does not automatically mean they are not members of the college. Some surgeons will not indicate their membership because they would have too many initials after their name if they included all of their degrees. Please see Table 2 for the training of doctors who manage pelvic floor disorders.

Surgeons in either urology or obstetrics and gynecology have to pass a written and oral examination after completing residency training in order to become board certified in either of these specialties. We both know experienced urogynecology and urology colleagues who have not completed fellowship training in FPMRS because no such training existed when they became board certified. These individuals are skilled surgeons. Thus, fellowship training in FPMRS is not a necessity, but it is an indication of additional expertise in the areas of pelvic dysfunction and pelvic reconstructive surgery. Board examination for FPMRS will start in June of 2013.

Table 2. Training of doctors who manage pelvic floor disorders

Specialty of surgeon (by self-designation)	Type of residency training and duration	Fellowship training and duration	Which American board of specialty they belong to
Urologist	Urology, 5 years	None	ABU
Gynecologist	Obstetrics and Gynecology, 4 years	None	ABOG
Urogynecologist	Obstetrics and Gynecology, 4 years	Variable: some do not have fellowship training, others have between 1 to 3 years	ABOG
Female Urologist	Urology, 5 years	1 or 2 years	ABU

Female Pelvic Medicine and Reconstructive Surgeon	Either of the above specialties, 4 or 5 years	Urology, 2 years Gynecology, 3 years	Either or both ABU and ABOG

ABU = American Board of Urology
ABOG = American Board of Obstetrics and Gynecology

Experience and current surgical volume

If you're deciding between two surgeons, how do you decide which surgeon to choose? We will present two scenarios below to demonstrate how experience and surgical volume come into play. How do you choose between two surgeons if all else (i.e., credentials, board certification, and specialty) is equal between them.

Let's consider a couple of scenarios.

	Surgeon A	**Surgeon B**
Scenario 1	Experienced surgeon; currently performs 3 surgeries every year	Experienced surgeon; currently performs 300 surgeries every year
Scenario 2	Inexperienced surgeon; currently performs 100 surgeries every year	Experienced surgeon currently performs 10 surgeries per year

If the type of surgery you are going to have is intricate or requires specialized training, then we would recommend that you choose a surgeon who is regularly in the operating room. For scenario 1, we would recommend you go with surgeon B. Why? Surgery is a lot like performing a violin solo in front of large audience. In order to play the piece flawlessly, you have to practice over and over again and then be able to perform on stage without making any mistakes.

Scenario 2 is a little tougher. To clarify, by inexperience, we do not mean chronologically young. We both know numerous talented young surgeons. By inexperienced surgeon, we mean one who does not routinely perform the specific type of surgery you need even though he/she is of the same specialty. For scenario 2, we would recommend you go with surgeon B.

When you have found two potential surgeons and believe that one could be your future surgeon, you must do your homework before arriving for the initial consultation visit. Go on the Internet and use a search engine (Google, Yahoo, etc.) and research the condition you have. Arm yourself with as much information as you can and write down any questions that come to mind. To help you, in Chapter 12, we have listed important questions that you should ask your potential surgeons. Although by doing this research, we don't expect you to obtain an MD degree, we do want you to know pertinent information before you speak to your potential surgeon. Try to know the names of the one or two surgeries for the type of condition that you have. Also, know a few answers to basic questions such as, "What are the complications of surgery X?" or "What condition does surgery X treat?" This way, when you are talking to your potential surgeon, you will be able to better assess their answers and you will also be more conversant with them.

Trust Your Instincts

We both have heard the expression "I would take skill over personality any day when it comes to my surgeon." We are here to tell you that you shouldn't have to choose one over the other. You can find a great technical surgeon who also has a good bedside manner.

Besides, inquiring about his/her qualifications and technical experience, you should trust your instincts. Once you arrive at a doctor's office with your list of questions, pay attention to how the surgeon makes you feel when you're talking to him or her. Does he or she maintain eye contact with you? Does he/she sit down and give you his or her undivided attention? Is he or she confident in the way he/she answers your questions? Is he or she honest in his or her answers? Every surgery has the potential for complications. Even the best surgeon in the world has had complications in his/her career. The potential surgeon should be truthful about his or her complication rate. You don't want an overconfident surgeon, but at the same time, you don't want one that is not sure of his or her abilities in the operating room or one that waivers in his or her decisions. No two surgeries are exactly alike. Surgeries can be fast-paced, and right decisions have to be made quickly. Does the surgeon you are speaking to give you the impression that he or she can do that? Does your surgeon treat complications of other surgeons? This can be an indicator of technical expertise and high surgical skill. Be sure to take notes of important information that you learn at these consultation visits.

The Down-There Diet

What you eat affects your health. Throughout this book, you will encounter dietary recommendations that will have a very important impact on your pelvic health. These diets differ in specific nuanced ways, according to whether you have irritable bowel syndrome or incontinence, for example. But all of them are similar in some general ways.

In a nutshell, the Down There diet is as follows:

- High fiber
- Low salt
- Low oxalate (chapter five)
- Low fat
- Low in refined sugars
- Few if any processed foods
- Low in meat
- High in grains, fruits, and vegetables
- Low in dairy

We are not talking about portions sizes, but think in moderation. We are not recommending strict food combinations, but use the list above as a frame of reference.

The Bottom Line

If you have followed the guidelines that we have discussed, then probably you have found the right surgeon for you. In the chapters that follow, you will find reminders about your anatomy and how to choose the best doctor for your situation. Keep in mind that, at times, taking in all this information can feel like a daunting task. So we recommend using the book as a guide whenever you have a question about your gynecologic or urologic health. Now's let's get started!

Chapter Two

When It Gets Wet Down There:
How to Control Urinary Incontinence

For the past several years, 39-year-old Sandra has been leaking urine every time she coughs, sneezes, or goes for a run. An active, busy mother of three children, she is beyond frustrated, annoyed, and embarrassed by her situation. Since the delivery (all three births were vaginal) of her last child who weighed nine pounds, she has noticed an increase in her symptoms, never mind her self-consciousness about the odor often accompanying the leakage. But one of the most concerning new symptoms is the leaking of urine during sexual intimacy.

At first, Sandra wore a panty liner to help her cope with the symptoms, but over the past nine months (her baby is now almost a year old), she must use heavy pads that have to be changed multiple times each day. Like most women, Sandra was reluctant to approach her doctor. When she finally summoned the courage to say something to her Ob/Gyn, her doctor prescribed medicine that was supposed to make her bladder less overactive. However, after several weeks, Sandra's urine was again leaking through the pads; the medicine did not help at all. Sandra had also tried Kegel exercises, intermittently and without success. What many practitioners don't tell women is that Kegels seldom work unless women do the exercises vigilantly several times daily for several months; without that kind of repetition, the pubococcygeus (PC) muscles cannot rebuild or strengthen.

Making her condition even more uncomfortable, Sandra had also had several urinary tract and vaginal infections because when urine remains in the vagina, it triggers bacterial infection. By the time Sandra arrived in our offices, she was discouraged and despondent. In fact, Sandra was so unhappy she had recently started taking antidepressant medication.

Incontinence: An All-Too-Common Occurrence

Sandra is not alone. She and 15 million other American women suffer from urinary incontinence, or involuntary loss of urine, a very common condition for women that typically begins as women enter their forties, increasing after menopause. However, some women in their thirties and even some in their twenties experience incontinence. While some women leak only a few drops of urine, others leak a large volume, which is quite problematic and can be socially isolating, leading to low self-esteem and depression. Regardless of the volume of urinary leakage, the problem is of great concern to those who suffer from urinary incontinence. Let's take a look at how the problem develops.

How the Bladder and Urethra Work

The main purpose of the bladder, a muscular organ within the pelvis, is to store urine or liquid waste products made by the kidneys. The bladder is able to expand and contract, facilitating the storage of urine. Think of your bladder and urethra as a balloon that contains a stem used to inflate the balloon.

The urethra is a small tube, less than two inches long in women, located at the front of the vagina; it transports urine from the bladder to the outside of the body. The urethra contains the muscles of the sphincter (pronounced *sfink-ter*) that keeps urine inside the bladder until it is time to empty the bladder. Normally, during urination, the muscles in the wall of the bladder contract, forcing urine out of the bladder and into the urethra. At the same time, sphincter muscles surrounding the urethra relax, letting urine pass out of the body.

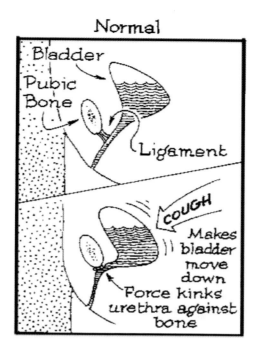

Using a balloon analogy, air will remain in a balloon as long as the stem is pinched off, or occluded. However, if the balloon builds up too much pressure, air will leak out. Also, if the stem is not completely compressed, any added pressure to the balloon will cause leakage of air. This is exactly what happens to the bladder and the urethra when incontinence occurs: either the bladder muscles suddenly contract or the sphincter muscles are not strong enough to hold urine back.

The sacral nerves, which are located near the tailbone, control the bladder and the muscles related to urinary function. If the brain and sacral nerves don't communicate correctly, the nerves can't tell the bladder to function properly. Or the bladder may be telling the brain that it is full when it is not. This communication problem can lead to symptoms of overactive bladder.

Common Causes of Incontinence

- Medications, especially diuretics (water pills) and drugs with caffeine
- Neurological disease such as multiple sclerosis, diabetes, Parkinson's disease, and dementia
- Urinary tract infection or other causes of bladder irritation
- Tumors, foreign bodies, and other abnormalities in the bladder such as bladder cancer
- Pregnancy or recent delivery, or history of traumatic childbirth

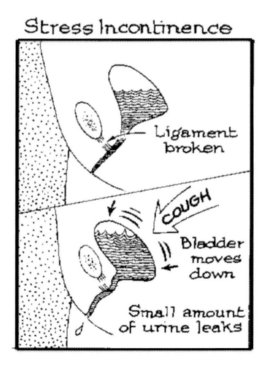

Stress Incontinence

Stress Incontinence

Stress incontinence has no relationship to emotional stress. Stress incontinence refers to the stress or added pressure that is placed on the bladder that overcomes the sphincters in the urethra and results in the leakage of small amounts of urine that occurs when the patients cough, sneeze, lift heavy objects, or even laugh. Sometimes patients mistakenly think that the term "stress incontinence" comes from the fact that they are stressed out and that is the reason they are having incontinence. This is a myth.

Let's go back to the balloon analogy: when too much pressure is placed on the body of the balloon (the bladder), the stem of the balloon or the sphincter in the urethra opens and allowing urine to escape.

Stress incontinence is usually caused by childbirth when babies pass through the birth canal and stretch all the muscles and ligaments in the pelvis, including the vaginal canal, which then weakens the support mechanisms of the bladder and the urethra. The more children a woman has by vaginal delivery, the greater the likelihood of developing stress incontinence because these muscles are out of place, are weak, and are unable to contract as quickly and effectively as they did before childbirth. With the bladder and the urethra out of place, any additional stress on the bladder will prevent the muscles in the urethra or sphincters from adequately compressing the urethra, causing urine to leak out of the bladder.

What You Can Do

The best way to prevent stress incontinence is to strengthen the muscles of the urethra and pelvis through regular and correctly done Kegel exercises. Another nonmedical solution is to train yourself to go to the restroom on a regular basis, so you can keep the bladder from getting too full. Keeping the urine volume in the bladder at a reduced level will help control incontinence. See below for more treatment options.

Some women will experience mild stress incontinence just before their menstrual period, when their estrogen levels naturally decrease. This decrease in estrogen lowers the sphincter pressure around the urethra and decreases the blood flow, leading to stress incontinence. Usually this mild stress incontinence that occurs before a woman's period lasts only a day or two and does not require treatment.

> Have you ever heard of the saying "I laughed so hard I peed my pants"? Many women think this situation is normal, but it is not. When laughter causes one to pee, it's another example of stress incontinence.

In addition, as women age and leave their childbearing years, the decrease in estrogen begins to cause changes to the vagina. When the ovaries cease to produce estrogen at menopause, even more pronounced changes occur in the vagina. Specifically, the decrease in estrogen triggers a decrease in blood supply to the vaginal tissues, which can result in vaginal atrophy or drying of the vaginal lining as well as atrophy of the urethra lining. Not only does vaginal atrophy result in urinary tract infections, sexual dysfunction, and vaginal infections, it also causes urinary incontinence.

Camille, a sixty-five-year-old woman, stopped having menstrual periods 15 years ago. Since then, she has experienced typical vaginal dryness and recently pain during intercourse. When she consulted her Ob/Gyn, he diagnosed her with vaginal dryness related to estrogen deficiency, and she was treated with a topical estrogen cream, which rapidly decreased her incontinence. Clearly, age is a factor with urinary incontinence. The exact changes that occur with aging that promote stress incontinence are not entirely known. But certainly hormonal changes and general stretching and laxity of the all the ligaments and muscles throughout the body as well as in the pelvis are contributing factors. Although there is nothing that can absolutely reverse these effects of aging, women can be proactive and maintain a healthy weight, avoid or stop smoking, and increase fiber in the diet (to avoid or decrease constipation)—all these actions will help relieve the stress associated with incontinence.

Besides childbirth, the most common cause of stress incontinence is any medical condition that is associated with an increase in abdominal pressure such as obesity, smoking (along with chronic coughing that typically accompanies smoking), and constipation. Any condition (e.g., emphysema) or activity (e.g., lifting something heavy) that increases intra-abdominal pressure (i.e., straining) makes an already battered and weak urethra susceptible to leakage of urine. Prolonged constipation leads to stool impaction in the rectum. Since the full rectum is in close proximity to the bladder, it can push on the bladder, irritate it, and lead to incontinence.

Finally, neurologic conditions, such as Parkinson's disease and Alzheimer's disease, surgery or radiation of the pelvis, and some medications that relax the sphincters in the urethra can be associated with stress incontinence.

Urge Incontinence or Overactive Bladder

"When you gotta go, you gotta go!" Unfortunately, many women are familiar with this popular saying. Urge incontinence or overactive bladder occurs when the bladder contracts without the owner's permission. This results in the situation that "when you gotta go, you gotta go!" Women with urge incontinence have a sudden, compelling desire to urinate that is difficult or impossible to defer. Women with urge incontinence have urgency of urination, urge incontinence, frequency of urination, and nocturia or nighttime voiding. Those who have urge incontinence will usually lose large volumes of urine all of a sudden with little or no warning time from the first urge to urinate to the compelling need to empty the bladder. A common scenario is when women do toilet mapping—when they know the location of most bathrooms around their town—so that if they are out and about, they can stop at a toilet just in case. Another common situation is when a woman returns home; as the key goes into the lock, the bladder starts to contract, and she is leaking urine before she has a chance to sit on the toilet.

Technically, there is an overactive bladder-wet and an overactive bladder-dry. The wet version is interchangeable with urge incontinence. Overactive bladder-dry means the person has to go to bathroom too many times, but there is no associated leakage.

To put this in perspective, women usually experience a 15-to 30-minute period between the first urge to go to the bathroom and the need to urinate. Those with overactive bladder often have a warning time that is just a few seconds, if any. Unlike stress incontinence, which results in small volumes of urine, urge incontinence makes the bladder contract and empty its entire contents all at once. As a result, panty liners or perineal pads will not be adequate to prevent the urine from going through the undergarments to the clothing. Sometimes, the only solution is to wear a diaper. Needless to say, this leads to discouragement, despondency, and the significant expense of adult diapers, the cost of which is not reimbursed by most insurance companies. (You can see why adult pads and diapers are part of a billion-dollar industry!)

A common cause of urge incontinence is inappropriate bladder contractions, often related to abnormal nerve signals. Certain medications such as diuretics or emotional states such as anxiety can worsen this condition. A complete list of medications that can potentially cause incontinence is shown in Table 1. Also, keep in mind that certain foods and fluids such as caffeine, tea, and artificially sweetened drinks also act as bladder irritants and can trigger the bladder to contract.

Some medical conditions, such as hyperthyroidism and uncontrolled diabetes, can also lead to or worsen urge incontinence. Urinary tract infections, emotional stress, or brain conditions such as Parkinson's disease or stroke also can trigger urge incontinence. Tumors of the bladder can cause the symptoms of frequency and urgency. Overactive bladder can be a complication of pelvic, bladder, or bowel surgery. Sometimes sutures or mesh from previous surgeries can erode into the bladder, causing overactive bladder symptoms. In addition, certain medical conditions are associated with overactive bladder, including fibromyalgia, a rare condition of muscle pain and fatigue; depression and anxiety; and irritable bowel syndrome, a common problem associated with cramping abdominal pain, bloating, and diarrhea or constipation (see Chapter Five on pelvic pain). However, the most common reason for overactive bladder and urge incontinence is idiopathic. In other words, something has gone wrong in the brain's ability to signal to bladder and vice versa.

Resource: For those who have urinary incontinence, we highly recommend the National Association For Continence, *www.nafc.org*. This non-profit website is dedicated to improving the quality of life of women with urinary incontinence.

Table 1. **Medications Causing Incontinence**

ANTIHYPERTENSIVE MEDICATIONS	Prazosin (Minipress), terazosin (Hytrin), doxazosin (Cardura), alpha-methyldopa (Aldomet), reserpine (Diupres, Hydropres)
DIURETICS	Furosemide (Lasix) or hydrochlorothiazide (Diuril), bumetanide (Bumex), spironolactone (Aldactone), theophylline
ANTIPSYCHOTIC DRUGS	Thioridazine, chlorpromazine (Thorazine), haloperidol (Haldol), and clozapine (Clozaril)
ANTIANXIETY DRUGS	Diazepam (Valium), alprazolam (Xanax), clonazepam (Klonopin)
ANTIDEPRESSANTS	Fluoxetine (Prozac), escitalopram (Lexapro), bupropion (Wellbutrin), sertraline (Zoloft), nortriptyline (Norpramin), benztropine (Congentin),
ANTI-PARKINSONISM DRUGS	Levodopa/carbidopa (Sinemet), ropinirole (Requip), pramipexole (Mirapex) ,

ANTIHYPERTENSIVE ACE INHIBITOR MEDICATIONS	Enalapril/hydrochlorothiazide (Vaseretic), enalapril (Vasotec), benazepril (Lotensin), fosinopril (Monopril), lisinopril (Zestril)
SEDATIVES AND SLEEPING PILLS	lorazepam (Ativan), diazepam (Valium), flurazepam (Dalmane), Eszopiclone (Lunesta), zolpidem (Ambien)
NARCOTICS AND PAINKILLERS	codeine (OxyContin), morphine (MS-Contin), oxycodone (Oramorph)

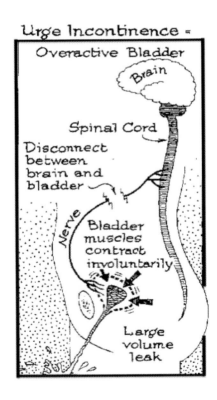

Urge Incontinence = Overactive Bladder

Mixed Incontinence

When women experience both stress and urge incontinence, the condition is referred to as mixed incontinence. It's very common for women to experience symptoms of both urge and stress incontinence. Usually, one type is more bothersome than the other. For example, a woman may mostly suffer from stress incontinence and only rarely be unable to reach the toilet in time. It is important for the patient's doctor to set appropriate expectations so the patient understands the options for treatment of mixed incontinence. If the patient has mixed incontinence but the stress component predominates, then surgery will help her. However, she should understand that surgery may not control the urge incontinence. Treatment for mixed incontinence may require a combination of modalities, including bladder training and medication after surgery.

Evaluation of Incontinence

It is important to define the type of incontinence that you have as the treatments vary for the different types of incontinence. First, you want to be seen by a doctor who has experience with the problem of urinary incontinence. This is usually a female pelvic medicine and reconstructive surgeon, a urologist, a gynecologist, or a urogynecologist, as all have some degree of training in the evaluation and treatment of urinary incontinence. Nurse practitioners and physical therapists with specialized training in women's health also can provide assistance for women with urinary incontinence. They help women identify the muscles in the pelvis and vagina and teach them how to strengthen these muscles in order to stop leakage. They also teach women how to control their urges so they can take control of their bladder. This is toilet training all over again. These therapists also educate about fluid management, reduction of foods that can aggravate the bladder, and behavioral changes that will allow women to have better control of their bladder for a longer period of time. The goal is not to leak or go to the bathroom for three to four hours. In the process of reaching this goal, women realize a higher quality of life.

The evaluation usually begins with a careful history. You can be of tremendous assistance to your doctor if you copy the bladder diary (at the end of this chapter) and document the fluid you consume, when you urinate, and the estimated fluid lost at various times of the day. To measure your urine output, you can use a special pan that fits over the toilet rim as shown in this photo.

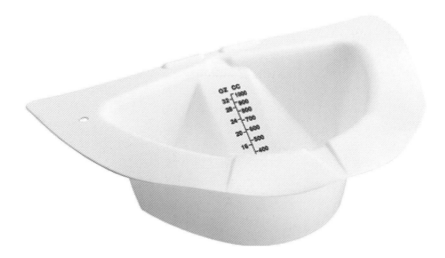

A voiding questionnaire plus a bladder diary can be invaluable to your physician and will aid and assist your doctor in making the correct diagnosis and customizing the proper treatment for your unique problem. Your pattern of voiding and urine leakage may suggest the type of incontinence you have. Then a general medical history is also completed that lists all your medications, previous treatments you have tried for your incontinence, recent surgery, and other medical illnesses such as diabetes, pulmonary diseases, and heart disease. The value of completing the bladder diary and the general health questionnaire is that it is often possible for you to begin treatment after your very first visit to the doctor's office.

Next is the physical examination. This usually consists of an abdominal examination and a pelvic examination. Your doctor will physically examine you for signs of medical conditions causing incontinence, including treatable blockages from bowel or pelvic growths. In addition, weakness of the pelvic floor leading to incontinence may cause a condition called prolapse, where the vagina or bladder begins to protrude out of your body. This condition is discussed in greater detail in Chapter Three. The doctor will also perform a brief neurologic examination checking for the nerve function in the pelvis and the lower extremities.

The doctor will usually examine you when your bladder is full and ask you to cough or bear down and pretend you are trying to have a bowel movement. The doctor will look for the loss of urine from the urethra during this part of the exam, which indicates stress urinary incontinence. Part of the physical exam is to measure the volume of urine the bladder can hold, or bladder capacity. After you urinate, the doctor will want to measure the remaining urine in the bladder or residual urine. This can be accomplished either by inserting a small tube or catheter into the bladder to measure the residual urine or by using a bladder ultrasound that can determine the amount of urine left in the bladder.

The minimal testing after the physical examination is a urine test or urinalysis. This very simple, inexpensive test is helpful to determine if there is a urinary tract infection, diabetes, bladder cancer, or kidney disease.

Women who have symptoms of both overactive bladder and stress incontinence may require a urodynamic test, which is used to measure the pressure within the bladder and the flow of urine from the bladder through the urethra. This test is also helpful in women with recurrence of their incontinence following previous incontinence surgery. Also, urodynamic testing is helpful for women who also suffer from multiple sclerosis, Parkinson's disease, or stroke.

Another test that may be performed in women with incontinence is a cystoscopy, which takes a picture of the interior of the bladder and the urethra, accomplished with the use of a small tube attached to a camera that is inserted through the urethra to observe the interior of the bladder and the urethra.

Change Your Life, Change Your Leakage

Women can make a lot of proactive steps to prevent if not reduce incontinence.

Avoiding Irritating Foods and Fluids

One of the first lines of defense is simply restricting certain fluids that are known bladder irritants such as coffee, tea, alcohol, and cola. And if urinary symptoms are a result of diet, you should see improvement 10 days after deleting the culprit. These fluids act like mild diuretics and increase the output of urine and naturally result in more frequent trips to the restroom. These drinks should also should be avoided in the evening or before bedtime, especially if you have a problem of nocturia or getting up at night to urinate.

Other foods such as citrus fruits, tomatoes, and almost every type of spicy food can irritate the bladder and cause it to spasm, resulting in urinary incontinence. Also, if you take diuretics or water pills, be sure to take them in the morning or early afternoon so that the increase urine output occurs before you go to sleep. A complete list of bladder irritants is shown in Table 2.

Following a Low-Acid Diet

A diet made up of foods low in acid may help some patients relieve the symptoms of overactive bladder. Low-acid fruits include blueberries, apples, grape juice, apple juice, pears, apricots, papayas, and watermelon. Kava (a coffee substitute) and noncitrus-herbal sun-brewed tea may alleviate the symptoms of urinary frequency and urgency. It's also helpful to take some supplements, including calcium carbonate co-buffered with ascorbate. Sugar itself is better than sugar-substitutes. Potatoes, fish, poultry, American cheese, cottage cheese, meats (avoid aged meats), bread (avoid sourdough and rye), rice, garlic, pasta, white chocolate, and frozen yogurt are also helpful in reducing urinary symptoms.

Table 2. Bladder Irritants

Apples	Mayonnaise
Apple juice	Nutrasweet
Cantaloupes	Peaches
Carbonated beverages	Pineapple
Chilies/spicy foods	Plums
Chocolate	Strawberries
Citrus Fruits	Tea
Coffee (including decaffeinated)	Tomatoes
Cranberries	Vinegar

Grapes   Artificially sweetened drinks
Guava
Vitamin B complex

Change your urinating habits—Bladder Retraining

Bladder retraining is another treatment option. Bladder retraining works to slowly increase the amount of urine the bladder can hold so that the intervals between peeing are longer. The average adult should urinate every two to four hours during the day and get up no more than once at night to urinate. Retraining the bladder is like reprogramming your bladder to contract at larger volumes and at more regular, predictable intervals so that you don't have sudden, unpredictable frequent leaks. This approach is easily accomplished by avoiding the first urge to urinate and attempting to increase the time interval in 15-minute increments on a weekly basis. You may even consider keeping a bladder diary (see sample diary at the end of this chapter) to track how often you use the rest room; if you find you have been going every 45 minutes during the day, you should try to increase that interval to an hour. By doing so, you can retrain your bladder to hold a greater volume of urine and slowly increase the time interval and the bladder capacity toward a normal level of three to four hours. If you note that increasing the time between voiding becomes uncomfortable, then back off and simply go when you need to relieve yourself.

We know it is difficult to remember to urinate at a set interval without a reminder. There are vibrating watches that can be programmed to vibrate at regular intervals. Some women use reminder watches not only for timed voiding, but for taking medication, checking blood sugar, carpool schedules, etc. These vibrating watches are available from National Incontinence (http://www.nationalincontinence.com/).

Timed Voiding

Another behavioral modification is "timed voiding," which consists of setting up a schedule of times to urinate. This schedule is determined by your personal habits and does not attempt to increase how long you can wait before having to urinate or to teach you to resist the urge to urinate. Helpful reminders include wristwatches with alarm settings that prompt you to urinate even when you don't have the desire to urinate. A simplified schedule might be to urinate before you get into the car to go on a trip. Then urinate as soon as you reach your destination or before you sit down for a meal or before you attend a movie or a function where you don't want to have to get up and leave to go the restroom. An effective bladder training program is shown at the end of this chapter.

You Can Strengthen Your Muscles!

Kegel exercises, named after Dr. Arnold Kegel, the gynecologist who identified the exercises in 1948 for the purpose preparing the pelvic muscles for childbirth, are now a multipurpose means of conditioning your muscles down there and preventing incontinence. Today we teach our patients to do "Turbo" Kegel exercises to treat urinary incontinence and accidental bowel leakage (which you will learn about in Chapter Seven). Any woman can perform these exercises at any time and at no cost.

Kegel exercises strengthen the muscles or sphincters that help control the urethra. When these muscles are weak, it is easier to develop urinary incontinence. These exercises, which can be done almost anywhere, can also delay and sometimes prevent pelvic organ prolapse, which is a condition when the pelvic organs descend and bulge into your vagina (see Chapter Three).

How to Do Turbo Kegels

The first step in learning how to do Kegels is to identify your pelvic floor muscles and learn how to contract and relax them. During the pelvic exam, we always ask our patients to show us a Kegel exercise while we have two examining fingers in the vagina. We often see their faces turn red, veins in the face appearing, the thighs try to close, the buttocks muscles quiver, and abdominal muscles contract—without any contraction of the muscles around the vagina. What does this mean? That despite the squeezing, a woman is demonstrating zero Kegel capacity.

The good news is that you can learn to identify the proper pelvic muscles by trying to stop the flow of urine while you're going to the bathroom. The other technique is using the muscles you use to stop from passing gas at a social gathering!

You can identify the correct muscles by simply inserting one or two fingers into your vagina and then trying to contract the muscles around your finger or fingers. After you have done this several times with the finger in the vagina, you can practice the exercise without having the necessity of inserting a finger.

After you've identified your pelvic floor muscles, contract these muscles and hold the contraction for three seconds then relax for three seconds. Repeat this exercise ten times. After you can hold your contraction for three seconds, try for six seconds, and then for 10. Ideally, we recommend that you do your Kegels at 7 reps, 7 sets per day, 7 times per week. That may sound like a lot, but one set takes about a minute, so we are recommending 7, 7-minute sets each week. The exercises will get easier the more often you do them. If you are doing the exercises correctly, you will feel like you are tightening your vagina and your rectum at the same time. You might make a practice of fitting in a set every time you do a routine task, such as sitting in your car at a red light, sitting at your desk, or during commercial breaks while watching TV. The beauty of Kegel exercises is that you can do them anytime and anywhere.

Unfortunately, results are not immediate, so don't expect to notice a change in your incontinence the first time you do these exercises. However, you will most likely notice a positive change within four to six weeks, and definitely a change within eight to twelve weeks. You will notice less frequent urine leakage, more sensation in your pelvic area, and possibly increased sexual responsiveness, especially reaching orgasm. The stronger your pelvic floor muscles, the more sexual pleasure you can expect. This was an accidental "side effect" discovered by Dr. Kegel. He heard back from his patients about these sexual benefits. As with any other kind of physical activity or exercise, you need to make Kegel exercises a lifelong practice to reap lifelong rewards.

The three most common mistakes we see in our practices when it comes to Kegel exercises are the following: (1) The wrong muscles are being trained/contracted; (2) women get bored or stop performing the exercises; and (3) the Kegels are not done regularly enough: strive for at least 7 reps, 7 sets, 7 times per week.

Devices That Help with Kegels

For those women who have trouble doing Kegel exercises or cannot identify the muscles in the pelvis that need to be contracted, biofeedback training or electrical stimulation may help. In a biofeedback session, a nurse, technician, or physical therapist with experience in pelvic floor or women's clinical specialist (WCS) will either insert a small monitoring probe into your vagina or place painless adhesive electrodes on the skin outside your vagina or rectal area. When you contract your pelvic floor muscles, you'll see a measurement on a monitor that lets you know whether you've successfully contracted the right muscles. You'll also be able to see how long you hold the contraction.

A number of different devices are available to help women identify their pelvic floor muscles and boost the intensity of the Kegel exercises themselves.

Step Free Vaginal Cones (available from National Incontinence (http://www.nationalincontinence.com/) consist of weighted cones that are easily inserted into the vagina, and the muscles are contracted to prevent the cones from falling out of the vagina.

Vaginal Cones

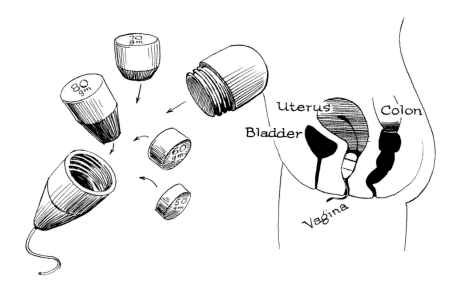

These cones are available in various weights and sizes, and women can perform the Kegel exercises with the cones in place. By gradually increasing the weight of the cone, a woman progressively increases the strength of her muscles. Again, exercising your pelvic floor with a pelvic floor exercise device offers biofeedback and adjustable resistance (depending on the device you chose).

Another device, the Kegelmaster, available from www.kegelmaster. com, is a plastic device shaped liked a dildo and is designed to strengthen vaginal tone and the muscles in the pelvis using dynamic progressive resistance, which results in improvement in bladder control. The device has an adjustable spring mechanism that allows you to control the degree of resistance against which your pelvic muscles contract. With increase in pelvic muscle strength, you progressively tighten the spring mechanism to maintain a level or resistance that continues to improve the strength and tone of the muscles in the vagina and results in improvement in incontinence. Just a comment here: Many patients mistakenly believe that Suzanne Somers' ThighMaster helps them do Kegel exercises. This is false!

When there is weakness or lengthening of the ligaments or pelvic support structures, a pessary can be inserted. This ring-shaped device made of rubber, plastic, or silicone that is similar in size and shape to a diaphragm can be easily inserted by a doctor (or by the woman herself if she is willing) and removed periodically for cleaning.

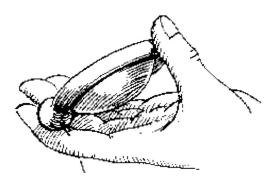

The two most commonly used pessaries are the ring with support and the Gellhorn. The ring with knob support is designed to treat stress urinary incontinence by providing additional support to the urethra during times of stress (coughing, laughing, etc.). The pessaries used for treating stress incontinence are not uniformly effective. More commonly, however, pessaries are used for treating prolapse (see Chapter Three).

Pessaries are especially recommended for women who have prolapse and/or stress incontinence and do not desire to have the condition repaired surgically. Pessaries are also used when symptoms of pelvic organ prolapse and urinary incontinence are mild. For example, if a woman has incontinence only during high-impact exercise, she can insert a pessary prior to exercising and remove it when she is finished. For young women who have prolapse or incontinence during pregnancy or in those who have not finished having children, a pessary is a nonsurgical, temporary solution until they have completed their family.

Women can have sexual intercourse with their pessary in place, depending on the type of pessary that is being used, but they cannot insert a diaphragm, which is used as a barrier method of birth control, while wearing a pessary. See Chapter Three for further details about pessaries.

Medications

Women whose incontinence does not improve with diet and Kegel exercises often resort to medication or surgical therapy. Before considering surgery, most doctors, including both of us, recommend that women try certain medications. Medications are particularly helpful in women with overactive bladder who have symptoms of frequency and urgency.

These medications are often referred to as bladder relaxants and are called anticholinergic medications because of the way they work on the body. These drugs relieve the symptoms of frequency and urgency by relaxing the muscles in the bladder. The most common overactive bladder medications include the following:

- Oral: Ditropan (oxybutynin), Detrol (tolterodine), Toviaz (fesoterodine), Enablex (darifenacin), Vesicare (solefenacin), Sanctura (trospium)
- Patch: Oxytrol (oxybutynin transdermal)
- Gel: Gelnique (oxybutynin gel)

The most common side effects of these drugs are dry mouth, constipation, and blurred vision. Other less common side effects include a faster heart rate, flushing, drowsiness, confusion, or memory loss. The side effects of confusion and memory loss are more common in the very elderly, and the newer anticholinergic medications are less likely to produce these problems.

One important note: many women who suffer from depression and are being treated with antidepressant medicines, including Zoloft and Paxil (see list of medications at the end of the chapter), sometimes develop incontinence as a side effect. The medicines, while helpful in relieving symptoms of depression, can impair the ability of the bladder to contract. Some medicines can also dull your awareness of the need to go to the bathroom.

However, one drug in particular, imipramine (Tofranil), sometimes is used to treat mixed urinary incontinence because of its bladder-relaxing effects as well as its urethral-contracting effects. Imipramine is not approved by the FDA for mixed urinary incontinence. This drug has been very effective in treating bedwetting in children and has been mildly effective in treating mild stress incontinence and overactive bladder.

Duloxetine is a drug that once showed promise for the treatment of stress incontinence. The drug was approved in Europe in 2004 but did not pass FDA approval in the United States for distribution to the public. The clinical trials certainly showed effectiveness in treating stress incontinence; however, the side effects included nausea and a slight link to suicide, prompting the manufacturers to withdraw their application from the FDA.

In postmenopausal women, topical estrogen creams inserted into the vagina have been used to treat the symptoms of both stress incontinence and the symptoms of overactive bladder. Estrogen increases the blood supply to the urethra and vagina and also increases the thickness of the lining of the vagina or vaginal mucosa. Estrogens have been used alone in women who demonstrate thinning or atrophy of the vaginal lining or in combination with anticholinergic medications. The results are certainly favorable for those women with mild stress incontinence and mild symptoms of overactive bladder. Estrogens are effective in postmenopausal women who are undergoing vaginal surgery as four to six weeks of topical estrogens will improve the thickness of the vaginal mucosa, making the surgical dissection easier, and will prevent breakdown of the tissues in the postoperative period.

Surgery for Stress Incontinence

Surgery is indicated primarily for the treatment of stress urinary incontinence. The procedures have undergone modification over the past two decades. A few years ago, surgical correction consisted of a major procedure requiring general anesthesia, hospitalization, and weeks or months to fully recover from the procedures. Now the procedures can be done on a minimally invasive basis in the doctor's office or ambulatory surgery center. These minimally invasive procedures, which take less than 20 minutes to perform, can be accomplished under local anesthesia or light sedation, and the patient can be discharged without a catheter. Throughout this book, we will briefly describe various surgical procedures while minimizing medical terminology. If you have questions about specific procedures listed on your surgical consent form, refer to the "Glossary of *Down There* Operations" at the end of the book for more detail.

Big Surgery with Long Incisions

Although uncommon, the open procedure for treatment of stress incontinence called the Burch, named after the gynecologist who first described the procedure, can be performed as a primary procedure to cure incontinence. However, today the Burch is performed more often as a secondary procedure when doctors are performing some other open abdominal surgery such as hysterectomy of sacrocolpopexy (see Chapter Three) since the long incision has already been made.

Tiny Incisions Using Slings

In 1996, a Swedish gynecologist developed the tension-free vaginal tape or TVT. This procedure consists of the placement of sling or hammock beneath the urethra through a small one-inch incision in the vagina. The sling is used to support the urethra and prevent the loss of urine when there is increased pressure in the abdomen with coughing, sneezing, or exercising. The sling acts like a hammock underneath the urethra to support it when the urethra moves downward during a cough or increase in intra-abdominal event.

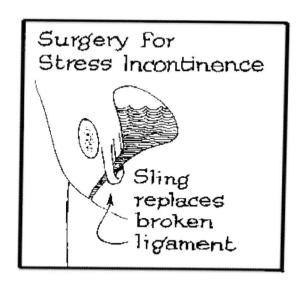

The location of the sling and the incision used to insert the sling are shown in the figure below.

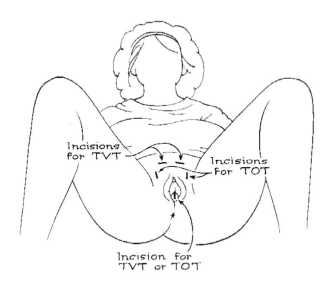

Today, the two most common types of slings are the TVT and the transobturator tape) (TOT) slings. Both of these slings use a polypropylene mesh tape placed underneath the urethra for support. TVT and TOT are safe and are not rejected by the body. The success rate for urethral slings approaches 90 percent. Complications are uncommon, but include over correction and urinary retention, urinary tract infection, pain, and exposure of the sling material into the vagina. If the sling is placed too tightly or it tightens, it can be loosened or cut. Another uncommon occurrence is exposure of the mesh. If this occurs, it can be remedied by removing the portion of the tape that has become exposed.

Insertion of Bulking Agents

Think of the urethra as a pipe or a tube that does not collapse and cannot hold the urine in place. By adding synthetic material made of Macroplastique or Coaptite, the diameter of the tube or the urethra can be narrowed and prevent the loss of urine. These injections around the urethra can be done under a local anesthetic in the doctor's office or in the ambulatory treatment center. The bulking procedure is best suited for women who do not wish to have a bigger procedure or who have multiple medical problems that make it difficult for them to undergo surgery. The procedure is also appropriate for women who have had other incontinence procedures such as a sling but still lose a small amount of urine and need to use pads. Often, the injection of the bulking agent will top off the leakage, and the women will become completely or almost completely dry.

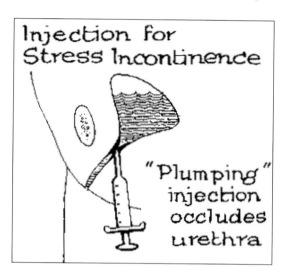

Injection for Stress Incontinence

"Plumping" injection occludes urethra

Radiofrequency Therapy

A recently FDA-approved treatment for stress incontinence makes use of the application of radiofrequency to the urethra and its junction with the bladder. This minimally invasive treatment can be accomplished in the doctor's office using a local anesthesia and oral medication for light sedation. The radiofrequency is delivered through a special catheter inserted into the urethra. The procedure takes approximately 30 minutes. The catheter is removed, and the woman leaves the office as soon as she can empty her bladder. Initial improvement may be followed by a return of symptoms for a few weeks and then slow improvement over the next six to eight weeks. The results show an improvement of approximately 50 percent in women who have had the radiofrequency treatment. The radiofrequency procedure is right for women with mild to moderate stress incontinence or for women who do not want to have one of the more invasive procedures.

However, this is a very new procedure, and we don't know the long-term effects of this yet.

Procedures or Surgery for Overactive Bladder

Most women with overactive bladder can be helped with medication and bladder exercises as mentioned previously. However, for those whose issues persist, surgery is also an option with a modest success rate. For women with small contracted bladders, adding segments of bowel to the bladder can increase the bladder capacity. This procedure is seldom performed because of the significant complications that occur.

Botox for Overactive Bladder

Botulinum toxin, or Botox, can be used for more than erasing those wrinkles on your forehead or the "crow's feet" at the corner of your eyes. Botox can be injected into the bladder to calm the contractions and reduce the symptoms of frequency and urgency. Botox is indicated for overactive bladder for women who fail treatment with anticholinergic medication.

Botox works by relaxing the contraction of muscles in the bladder by blocking the excessive nerve impulses that cause the bladder to contract and thus relieve the symptoms of frequency and urgency. A portion of the bladder muscles are then paralyzed and can no longer contract, and so the bladder relaxes. It usually takes several days to two weeks to see symptomatic improvement, and the effects tend to last from three to six months. Most women require retreatment in six to nine months when the symptoms return. Success rates have been reported as high as 75 percent reduction in urgency and frequency symptoms. The most common adverse effects are not being able to empty the bladder completely and bladder infection.

Neurostimulation

Neurostimulation is an option for managing the symptoms of overactive bladder for people who have not found success with more conservative treatments such as behavioral therapy or medication. By stimulating the nerves below the spinal cord that control urination, relief from severe urgency, frequency, urge incontinence, and urinary retention can be achieved. Stimulation of these nerves, known as sacral neuromodulation, was FDA approved in 1997 for urge incontinence and in 1999 for significant symptoms of urgency and frequency.

Neurostimulation targets the bladder-spinal cord-brain communication problem by stimulating the nerves with mild electrical pulses. The outpatient procedure consists of surgical placement of a stimulating wire into the sacral opening and a neurostimulator device beneath the skin in the upper buttocks. Don't worry, this is far away from your spinal cord, and there is no chance of causing paralysis. The device can be modulated and even turned on or off by the woman using a programming device. Neurostimulation is a reversible treatment that can be discontinued at any time by turning off or removing the device. There are two available neurostimulators, and each has a battery life of five to nine years before needing to be replaced.

The potential side effects or complications of neurostimulation include implant site pain, skin irritation, infection, device problems, and lead (thin wire) movement. These conditions are generally treatable. And, of course, 100 percent will need reoperation for removal and replacement of the battery after it runs out.

Posterior Tibial Nerve Stimulation

Posterior tibial nerve stimulation (PTNS) is a technique of electrical neuromodulation for the treatment of overactive bladder in patients who have not had success with diet and exercise. The tibial nerve located in each lower extremity is accessed using a fine needle inserted slightly above the ankle, and low-voltage electrical stimulation is delivered. The course of treatment is typically 12 weeks of 30-minute weekly sessions.

The treatment works by stimulating the posterior tibial nerve, which is derived from the same sacral nerves that control the bladder and muscles within the pelvis. Altering the function of the posterior tibial nerve with PTNS is believed to improve voiding function and control.

PTNS is a low-risk procedure. The most common side effects with PTNS treatment are temporary and minor, resulting from the placement of the needle electrode. They include minor bleeding, mild pain, and skin inflammation. The good news is that PTNS is a minimally invasive treatment that is easily accomplished in the doctor's office.

The Bottom Line

So what happened to Sandra? Sandra was found to have pure stress incontinence. She came to the hospital early one morning, and while she was under light sedation, we placed a TOT sling to support her urethra. The procedure took less than 20 minutes. Forty-five minutes after the procedure, she was able to urinate, and she was discharged and completely dry. Within four to six weeks, she began exercising and playing tennis, and did not need any pads or panty liners. She also stopped taking her antidepressant medication.

Her comment was, "Doctor, you gave me my life back. Thank you from the bottom of my heart."

The bottom line is this: Urinary incontinence is a common problem that impacts the quality of life of millions of American women. An evaluation is easily accomplished in the doctor's office, and help is available for nearly all women wearing diapers and using pads to avoid the embarrassing situation and to cure many who suffer from this condition. You don't have to depend on Depend™!

In the next chapter, you will read about another common and related problem down there—when your pelvic organs drop and bulge into the vagina.

BLADDER TRAINING PROGRAM

1. Begin a diary to record the times that you go to the bathroom.

2. Empty your bladder first thing in the morning.

3. Void throughout the day by the clock, not by how you feel. Start with voiding every two hours if you can. Initially, if this is too difficult, start with voiding every hour. Wait the full amount of time to urinate, and empty your bladder even if you do not feel the urge to. Empty at bedtime. And at night, go only if you awaken and find it necessary.

4. If you feel a strong urge before it is time to void, use the following urge suppression techniques:

    Stop. Do not rush to the bathroom. Think about anything but the toilet (what you made for dinner last night, what you are doing tonight, count backward by sevens from 100, etc.).

    Perform five quick pelvic floor muscle "squeezes" or Kegels, wait 10 seconds and repeat.

    Take three slow, deep breaths, concentrating on the inhale and exhale.

5. Once you are comfortable with this two-hour interval for five to seven days, increase it by 15 to 30 minutes.

6. Gradually increase the duration and frequency until you are voiding at a normal three-to four-hour interval.

7. Keep a diary twice a week to measure and document progress. Only measure the interval of your voids (times), and do not worry about voided volumes.

8. Be patient. It will take from six to 12 weeks to reach your goal. Don't get discouraged. You will have good and bad days. As you continue, you will notice more good days.

9. Keep your scheduled visits and bring your diaries.

10. Consider other treatment options if not effective in three to four weeks.

*Modified from http://familydoctor.org/familydoctor/en/diseases-conditions/urinary-incontinence/treatment/bladder-training-for-urinary-incontinence.html

Bladder Diary*

Your Daily Bladder Diary

This diary will help you and your health care team figure out the causes of your bladder control trouble. The "sample" line shows you how to use the diary.

Your name: _____

Date: _____

Time	Drinks		Trips to the Bathroom		Accidental Leaks	Did you feel a strong urge to go?	What were you doing at the time?
			How many times?	How much urine? (circle one)	How much? (circle one)	Circle one	Sneezing, exercising having sex, lifting, etc.
	What kind?	How much?					
Sample	Coffee	2 cups	✓✓	⊙ ○ ○ sm med lg	○ ⊙ ○ sm med lg	Yes (No)	Running
6–7 a.m.				○ ○ ○	○ ○ ○	Yes No	
7–8 a.m.				○ ○ ○	○ ○ ○	Yes No	
8–9 a.m.				○ ○ ○	○ ○ ○	Yes No	
9–10 a.m.				○ ○ ○	○ ○ ○	Yes No	
10–11 a.m.				○ ○ ○	○ ○ ○	Yes No	
11–12 noon				○ ○ ○	○ ○ ○	Yes No	
12–1 p.m.				○ ○ ○	○ ○ ○	Yes No	
1–2 p.m.				○ ○ ○	○ ○ ○	Yes No	
2–3 p.m.				○ ○ ○	○ ○ ○	Yes No	
3–4 p.m.				○ ○ ○	○ ○ ○	Yes No	
4–5 p.m				○ ○ ○	○ ○ ○	Yes No	
5–6 p.m.				○ ○ ○	○ ○ ○	Yes No	
6–7 p.m.				○ ○ ○	○ ○ ○	Yes No	

Use this sheet as a master for making copies that you can use as a bladder diary for as many days as you need.

Time	Drinks		Trips to the Bathroom		Accidental Leaks	Did you feel a strong urge to go?	What were you doing at the time?
			How many times?	*How much urine? (circle one)*	*How much? (circle one)*	*Circle one*	*Sneezing, exercising having sex, lifting, etc.*
	What kind?	*How much?*					
Sample	**Soda**	**2 cans**	✓✓	⊙ ○ ○ sm med lg	⊙ ○ ○ sm med lg	Yes (No)	**Running**
7–8 p.m.				○ ○ ○	○ ○ ○	Yes No	
8–9 p.m.				○ ○ ○	○ ○ ○	Yes No	
9–10 p.m.				○ ○ ○	○ ○ ○	Yes No	
10–11 p.m.				○ ○ ○	○ ○ ○	Yes No	
11–12 midnight				○ ○ ○	○ ○ ○	Yes No	
12–1 a.m.				○ ○ ○	○ ○ ○	Yes No	
1–2 a.m.				○ ○ ○	○ ○ ○	Yes No	
2–3 a.m.				○ ○ ○	○ ○ ○	Yes No	
3–4 a.m.				○ ○ ○	○ ○ ○	Yes No	
4–5 a.m.				○ ○ ○	○ ○ ○	Yes No	
5–6 a.m.				○ ○ ○	○ ○ ○	Yes No	

I used _____ pads today. I used _____ diapers today (write number).

Questions to ask my health care team: _____

_____

_____

_____

_____

*http://kegel-exercises.com/bladder_diary.pdf

Chapter Three

When More Than London
Bridge Is Falling Down:
Pelvic Organ Prolapse

Melissa is a 49-year-old woman who came to us for evaluation. She first noticed that something didn't feel right down there 14 months earlier. At first, she thought the problem was all in her head, but the sensation of heaviness and pressure in her vagina just didn't go away. Melissa described the feeling as if a tampon was stuck inside, even though she doesn't use tampons. She felt like something was loose and moving around. Melissa also told us that she has given birth to four children and recalled, "It took them a long time to sew me up down there." The feeling of pulling and heaviness worsened throughout the day, especially if she had been on her feet for hours at a time. Melissa also noticed that she had to go to the bathroom way too many times during the day and got up two or three times at night. Even though she did not have any leakage, she wore a panty liner just in case.

Then eight months ago, while showering, Melissa felt a bulge down there and immediately grabbed a hand mirror and noticed an orange-size lump protruding from her vagina. "Oh my gosh," she thought to herself, "Do I have cancer?" She made the next available appointment with her gynecologist who immediately diagnosed pelvic organ prolapse (POP) and sent her to see one of us in our clinic.

Pelvic organ prolapse is the term that doctors use to describe a number of problems that women can experience when their pelvic organs (uterus, bladder, rectum, or bowel) shift out of place, slip, and then fall from their normal position into the vagina. Heaviness and discomfort in the vagina are the most common symptoms that accompany POP. Often, patients will notice or feel a bulge or protrusion down there. Besides these common symptoms, some women may also experience pain in their pelvis or lower back, and some feel looseness in their vagina.

POP is so common that up to one out of every two women has or will develop this uncomfortable medical condition that can disrupt a woman's quality of life. That means 50 percent of women will encounter this condition at least once in their lifetime! For many women, mild to moderate POP is not painful, and some women may not show any symptoms until later in life.

The risk of prolapse does increase as women age. When women become menopausal, the lack of estrogen predisposes the connective tissues and muscles to laxity as well as the loss of collagen content and thinning because those tissues have estrogen receptors. And for reasons that are not yet understood, white and Hispanic women are more likely than black women to have symptoms of POP.

Why Am I Falling Apart Down There?

Three pelvic organs, the uterus, bladder, and rectum, are held in place by strong connective tissue that wraps around the cervix like a bandage. Like thick ropes, strong ligaments attach to this connective tissue bandage and suspend the uterus in the middle of the pelvis. These ropes are called the cardinal and uterosacral ligaments (see drawing on next page). The bladder sits on a flat shelf of connective tissue, which is suspended and attached to the sides of the pelvis like a hammock. This shelf is called the pubocervical septum. Similarly, a shelf of connective tissue separates and keeps the rectum and vagina next to each other but neighbors, like wall separators between cubicles. This is called the rectovaginal septum.

Suspension System

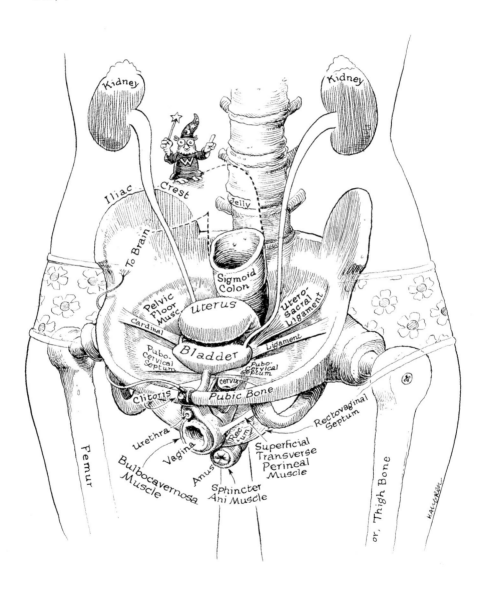

The three pelvic organs are held in place by these ropes and bandages. The ropes are, in turn, attached to large flat muscles, which are attached to the bones of the pelvis. When the muscles contract, the rope is taut. When the muscles relax, the rope becomes slack. When these pelvic floor muscles are strong and working well, they help keep the ligaments taut and thus suspend the pelvic organs in the middle of the pelvis.

The bowel is free-floating in the pelvis like Jell-O in a big glass bowl. It will slide into any area that has lost its strength and support. Therefore, we consider a bowel protrusion into the vagina an enterocele, or a true hernia.

After a woman pushes out a few little munchkins, the ropes can break, the bandages can rip, and the pelvic muscles may not work as well anymore. The pelvic organs gradually lose their support, slip, and then fall down the well, the vagina. Imagine a large bucket full of water hanging from a rope over the middle of a well. This is the normal ideal scenario where undamaged ligaments are supporting the weight of the pelvic organs. Now, imagine that instead of the rope, the bucket is suspended by a rubber band. The thinner the rubber band, the more the bucket sags. If the rubber band isn't able to hold up the bucket, it can snap at any moment, and the bucket will drop. I am sure you get the picture.

Prolapse is triggered by a combination of factors—the two biggest negative forces are traumatic childbirth and genetic predisposition. Women with genetic predisposition are not the only ones who get prolapse. Currently, there is no genetic test for prolapse, but you can assume that you have a genetic predisposition if your mom, sister, twin, especially first-degree relatives, had prolapse. Also, certain diseases such as spina bifida, Ehlers-Danlos, and bladder extrophy predispose a woman to getting prolapse.

While the baby is coming through the birth canal, it can stretch and tear the tissues, like a scissor cutting through your favorite satin bedsheets. As a result of the stretching and tearing, the tissue weakens, and nerves may get damaged. The body may not be able to repair the tissue and nerve damage and put it back in place just like it was before the baby was born. The resulting weakness and sagging becomes worse as a woman gets older. Over time, if the muscles are not rehabilitated and negative lifestyle forces are not reduced (i.e., straining, heavy lifting, constipation, obesity, smoking, coughing), the tissues will continue to worsen. Also, as mentioned before, age-related changes that take place especially from age 60 onward leading to thinning tissue, wrinkling skin, and muscle atrophy also contribute. The muscles that line the vagina and form the opening of the vagina also get stretched—all of which are weakened or damaged during childbirth.

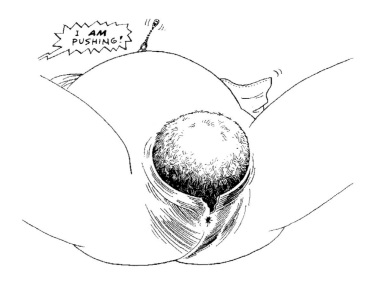

The pelvic organs are supported by a trampoline of muscles and connective tissues. Every time you strain, cough, and lift, it is as if a big teenager bounces up and down on your toddler's small trampoline. Eventually, the strings supporting the trampoline net begin to wear down and even break. Eventually, the muscles and connective tissues that hold the pelvic organs in place give way; and the uterus, bladder, rectum, or bowel can then drop into the vagina. The pelvic organs keep dropping lower and lower, until one day, they literally fall out of the vagina, and a bulge is seen or felt between the legs. Like fruit, a prolapse can come in different sizes, but the largest either one of us has ever seen was the size of a small watermelon (see drawing on the next page). The woman's complaint when she finally came to the office? "Doctor, something is not right down there!"

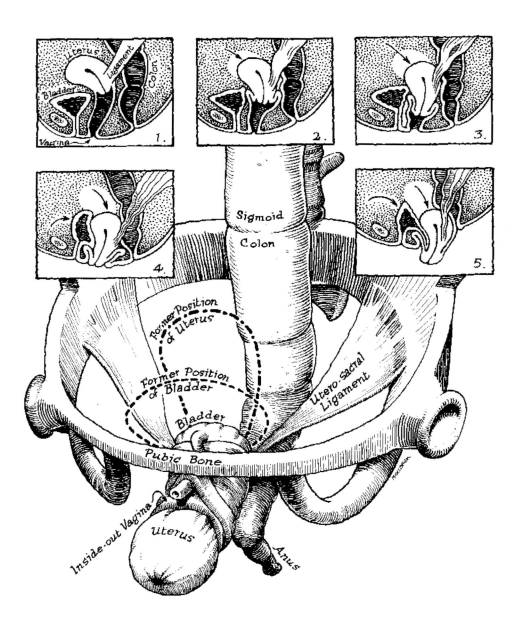

Are You Genetically Predisposed to Prolapse?

Family history and race are known risk factors. A pale-skinned, light-haired white woman whose mother and older sister had POP is at higher risk for POP than a dark-skinned African woman. A family history of prolapse and incontinence and white and Hispanic race seem to be risk factors.

Here is a list of other risk factors:

- Traumatic and multiple childbirths are two of the strongest risk factors for POP. A patient who was in labor for a long time, was unable to push out her large baby, and who then required forceps to pull out the baby, or who sustained a large tear in her vaginal tissues is often at high risk of POP and pelvic dysfunction in the future. Although the first vaginal birth has the greatest potential to cause damage, subsequent childbirths don't spare the tissues. A woman who has birthed six children through her birth canal does have a higher risk of POP than someone who has delivered only one baby.

- Aging and gravity both increase the toll on already weakened support of the pelvic organs. Add to this the effects of routine increases in the pressure inside the abdomen, and you've got even more reason to have POP. Lifestyle habits that chronically and repeatedly elevate the pressure inside of the abdominal cavity can make prolapse worse: a smoker who coughs several times every day or a sedentary, older woman who consumes little fiber, or a middle-age woman who has to strain hard because she is constipated.

- Anytime a woman lifts heavy objects that strain the muscles (lower abdomen and groin muscles, as well as the internal pelvic muscles), they can put excessive pressure on the pelvic organs. We both have had numerous patients who work in careers that require lifting of heavy objects. Postal workers, nurses and physical therapists, childcare providers, and factory workers all do heavy, repetitive lifting in their daily work.

How to Help Avoid POP

If one of our patients has surgery, we advise her to do no heavy lifting for a few weeks after surgery. Additionally, when she is ready to go back to work, we counsel her to use proper lifting technique, use mechanical assistance if working in a factory, and try to minimize lifting duties or be reassigned to less rigorous duties at work. Since a prolapse is like a hernia in the vagina, we suggest that you take precaution when doing any lifting of heavy items. Here are some suggestions to avoid straining your muscles:

1. Avoid lifting objects that are too heavy or awkward shaped.
2. Ask for help.
3. Use an assistive device (e.g., wheeled cart, handtruck, forklift).
4. Keep your feet shoulder width apart, and place one foot beside the object and the other foot behind the object so you can maintain balance.
5. Lift with your legs (not with your back—do not bend from the waist to lift objects). Bend at the knees, and keep your back nearly straight but in comfortable position.
6. Contract your pelvic muscles, buttocks, and abdomen as you lift and ease the load up instead of jerking it.
7. Carry the item close to your body.
8. Bend at the knees and reverse the above steps to deposit the object.

Prolapse and Bladder Issues

Too bad for us, science hasn't discovered a way to predict what urinary symptoms a woman will have based on the type and extent of her prolapse. We can show you four women who are the same age, same stature, and with the same exact POP, and each may complain of a different urinary symptom. For example, imagine four women who have prolapse. Each may have a different urinary problem that is bothersome to her: the first woman may have a constant urge to go the bathroom and frequents the toilet at least 10 times a day and knows the exact location of every bathroom in her town. A second woman may have no urgency to urinate, but she finds it difficult to start peeing, feels like she doesn't completely empty her bladder unless she has lain down for an hour before going to the toilet, and then has to lean forward to urinate. A third woman with the same exact prolapse may pee on herself every time she coughs, laughs, gets up from a chair, or bends down to pick up something. Finally, a fourth woman may have the exact same prolapse as the three women just described, but may have absolutely no urinary problems. Because of the diversity in symptoms and the complexity of POP, it is often necessary to perform urodynamic testing (see Chapter Two), which is used to measure the pressure within the bladder and the flow of urine from the bladder through the urethra; urodynamic testing allows customization of the treatment for each patient. One size dress doesn't fit all!

The Truth about Delivery

True or false: If all the pregnant woman in the country were not allowed to have vaginal childbirth (in other words, if the president of the United States signed a law that mandated all women in the United States to deliver their babies by Cesarean section), then nobody would develop POP. False! Although the number of women developing POP would be reduced, some women would still develop prolapse. Because there are multiple risk factors for prolapse, eliminating one of them (even though it may be a big one) won't prevent POP. Even cloistered nuns can develop POP!

It is also not accurate to assume that C-sections avoid all risks of prolapse. Cesarean section itself has risks. It is a major surgery, which can be associated with complications more often than vaginal childbirth. These include infection, bleeding, and injury to organs around the uterus. Women who have multiple C-sections also can develop life-threatening hemorrhage if their placenta fuses into the old cesarean scar and doesn't separate. The more C-sections a woman has had, the higher the chance that the placenta will be superglued to the womb. A baby going though the birth canal is a good thing. It does have advantages. Vaginally delivered babies are less likely to have breathing problems, can initiate breastfeeding with less difficulty, and can bond immediately with mom. Nevertheless, there are certain situations when a Cesarean section may be beneficial for the *down there* of the mother. Your obstetrician can be of tremendous assistance to help you weigh the risks and benefits of an elective Cesarean section.

Avoid Smoking—It May Be Hazardous to Your Pelvis

Okay, enough of the heavy. Let's talk about other things you can do to reduce your risk of POP. We all know that smoking is bad, and nicotine is addictive. Smoking leads to emphysema of the lung and is a risk factor for lung cancer. Smokers also have difficulty healing their tissues. Chronic smokers tend to cough a lot, and too much coughing is a strong risk factor for POP. Remember, every time you cough, you are placing increased pressure on your pelvic muscles and organs. Every cough stresses those ligaments and ropes holding that trampoline in place. With years of coughing, it is no wonder that the ropes give way and the trampoline breaks. There are also certain types of blood pressure medications, known as angiotensin-converting enzyme (ACE) inhibitors, including captopril and enalapril, whose side effect is dry cough. If you are experiencing these problems, you may want to ask your doctor to change your medication if it possible.

Diet High in Fiber

The typical American diet is low in fiber, which many of us know is a risk factor for colon cancer. It's also a risk for prolapse. To keep your colon and pelvic organs in healthy, strong shape, we recommend that you consume 35 grams of fiber daily. For example, if you consume three servings of fruit (9.3 grams); two servings of vegetables (8.7 grams); three servings of fiber-rich grains such as whole-wheat bread, brown rice, raisin bran cereal (16.5 grams); and 1 tablespoon of walnuts (1.1 grams), then your diet contains an adequate amount of fiber. A list of fiber-rich foods is provided in the box below.

- Choose more fresh fruits and vegetables:

    apples
    pears
    bananas
    potatoes
    blueberries
    prunes
    broccoli
    raisins
    Brussels sprouts
    pinach
    cantaloupe
    strawberries
    carrots
    sweet potatoes
    figs
    tomatoes
    oranges
    zucchini
    peaches

- Choose more whole-grain breads, pastas, and cereals:

    All-Bran
    oat bran
    barley
    oatmeal
    Bran Flakes
    pumpernickel bread
    brown rice
    Raisin Bran
    granola
    whole-grain breads

- Choose more dried beans, peas, nuts, and seeds (as tolerated):

  baked beans
  split peas
  lentils
  sunflower seeds
  peanuts
  walnuts
  soy products, such as tofu and textured vegetable
     protein

- Choose more snacks that are high in fiber:

  cereal mix with nuts and seeds
  fresh fruit
  fresh vegetables
  popcorn
  whole grain cereal
  yogurt with bran cereal

- Plan more vegetarian meals:

  bean and rice burritos
  beans and rice
  hummus and pita bread
  pasta with vegetables
  split pea or lentil soup
  vegetable stir fry

If you are unable to meet this recommendation through your food choices, then it's best to take a daily fiber supplement. If you find yourself sitting on the toilet for a long time conducting your business or you have developed a habit of reading an entire book or the whole Sunday edition of the newspaper in the bathroom because you are in there for so long, then you may be constipated. Adequate fiber intake and regular activity or exercise can relieve constipation and will promote regular soft bowel movements without putting strain on your pelvic floor muscles. Having said all that, be careful with taking too much fiber too fast. Your body will not like it, and you will get bloated and gassy. Always go slow and gradually increase until you reach a comfortable consistency of your bowel movements.

How Do I Get Rid of This Nuisance Down There?

When we see a patient who comes to us or has been referred to us for prolapse, we offer her several options for treatment depending on her situation. If the patient was sent to us by her primary care doctor or gynecologist because a small bulge in the vagina was noticed during the Pap smear, but doesn't have any other symptoms such as pressure, bulge, or sexual, urinary, or defecatory problems, then we advise her to do Kegel exercises, which we refer to as Turbo Kegels (see Chapter Two).

If the patient has mild prolapse and has symptoms related to urinating or defecating, then we will make recommendations to solve those problems, including modifying her diet, increasing daily fiber intake, and going to the bathroom about the same time each day (especially in the morning before leaving her home). For the urinary symptoms, we may recommend regular, timed-toileting or gradually waiting longer and longer between voids. In other words, we are going to suggest that she go through toilet training all over again (see Chapter Two). Additionally, women who have mild prolapse symptoms can benefit from Turbo Kegels.

The Quick Fix

If your prolapse is bothering you, then a pessary may be an acceptable option. Pessaries date back to ancient Egypt when healers performed various maneuvers to remedy the prolapsed womb. Many of the methods used in the past were not only unsuccessful, but they were also painful and bizarre. Women were hung upside down from their feet and bounced up and down so that the prolapse would disappear. Smoke was directed and hot oils were rubbed on the prolapse in an attempt to reduce it.

Another treatment included cupping the buttocks for hours in hopes that the prolapse would be sucked back in.

The more successful methods of treating prolapse came later by shoving large round objects, such as half a pomegranate, into the vagina to hold the pelvic organs in place. With all these seemingly barbaric treatments, is it any wonder that the women of today can't describe their symptoms and will suffer in silence for years before talking to a physician about their symptoms down there?

Thankfully, medical doctors finally realized that prolapse is a problem of the lack of support of the pelvic anatomy and began to invent different objects that could hold the pelvic organs in place by lodging the object into the vagina. Today, pessaries are made of soft rubbery material called silicone. The pessary is safe, nonallergenic, and resists infections. Pessaries come in various shapes and sizes, but the most commonly used pessary is called the ring with diaphragm.

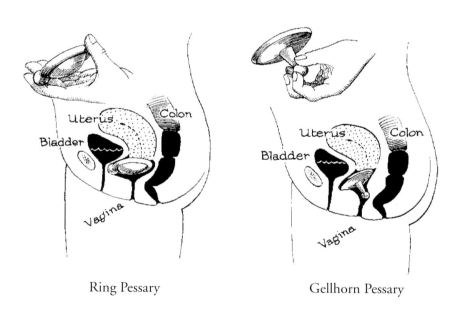

Ring Pessary · Gellhorn Pessary

The pessary is fitted and placed inside the vagina (this takes less than a minute), and it helps keep the pelvic organs in place. Although a pessary may lead to some shrinkage of the prolapse, it will not make the prolapse go away completely. The pessary keeps the prolapse from coming out. It is like a bandage on a cut. It doesn't fix the cut, but it does keep it covered and clean.

In a few circumstances, we would recommend a pessary over surgery. If a woman wishes to have future pregnancy and childbirth, there is no point to fix her prolapse surgically—because subsequent childbirth can undo the repair. Some women choose a pessary initially because of financial problems or if her schedule doesn't permit her to take an extended leave from her job to recover from surgery. Also, older women with other, complicated medical problems may choose a pessary instead of surgery.

A pessary may not be right for some women as their vagina may be too large and stretched out to hold one, and the pessary may pop right out as soon as she stands up, coughs, or strains. Also, women who have small contracted vaginas because of lack of estrogen or atrophy may also not be able to tolerate a pessary. Even though a pessary probably doesn't cause a vaginal infection, it can make the vagina produce more discharge and odor, which may not be acceptable for some women. After all, the pessary is a foreign body, and vaginas don't like things that are not natural or are foreign to be in there for long periods of time.

Some women do not feel comfortable having a pessary inside their vagina. The ring pessary (soft silicone) can be worn during sex, although some couples prefer to remove it before sex. Other pessaries, such as the Gellhorn, must be removed before sex. With these pessaries, sexual activity may be continued as long as a woman is able to remove and reinsert the pessary herself. Some women are unable or unwilling to do this. For them, regular visits (every three months) to the doctor is important in order to clean the pessary and to make sure that it has not caused any problems, such as a vaginal ulceration or erosion, difficulty with bowel movements, or development of urinary leakage. If you choose to insert and remove the pessary yourself, be sure to see your doctor once each year for a checkup so the vagina can be examined for any problems. In our practices, often we find that women with prolapse who are young, active, and/or who have severe POP are more likely to reject pessary as a treatment option for their prolapse. Nevertheless, for those women who are okay with all of the above, the pessary can be an effective non-surgical method to treat their prolapse symptoms.

Treating Your Prolapse

Indication for medical treatment of a prolapse is any symptom that is bothersome to the patient, including bulge, heaviness, pain, and urinary/ sexual or defecation problems. Surgically, there are two effective approaches to fix POP: an abdominal and/or a vaginal operation. If technology is added to traditional techniques of repair, then the same surgery can be achieved by a laparoscopic or a robotic technique, which is less invasive and leads to a faster recovery. If your surgeon chooses the abdominal route, then a horizontal, five-inch cut is made in the skin near the hairline just above the pubic bone, and the majority or all the operation is performed through this incision. Don't worry, your incision can be hidden beneath your bikini line.

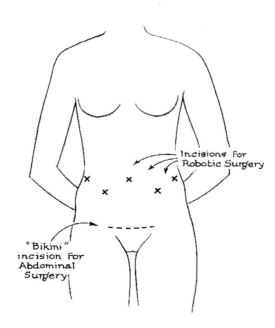

Abdominal Surgery

During the abdominal operation for POP, or abdominal sacrocolpopexy (A-SCP), either two rectangular pieces of synthetic mesh (two by five inches) or a Y-shaped piece of mesh is used to suspend the vagina to the sacrum (see Glossary of Operations for more detail). The back (rectovaginal septum) and front (pubocervical septum) of the vagina are sandwiched between the mesh and held in place with sutures. This sandwich of vagina and mesh, in turn, is suspended to the ligament over the sacrum by permanent sutures.

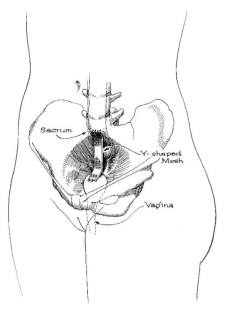

Sacrocolpopexy

The typical recovery period is six to eight weeks for this abdominal operation. You will not feel the attachment of mesh to your tailbone. The A-SCP operation is strong as well as resilient and long lasting. We have more than 50 years of scientific knowledge about the A-SCP operation. This surgery for POP truly has passed the test of time!

Vaginal Surgery

Another method of repairing your prolapse is by doing the entire operation through the vagina, which has the benefit of not making a single opening on your belly and leaving no scar. Because this surgery leaves no trace, some women prefer it.

Many women choose vaginal surgery because they will spend less time in the operating room, and it's a minimally invasive procedure.

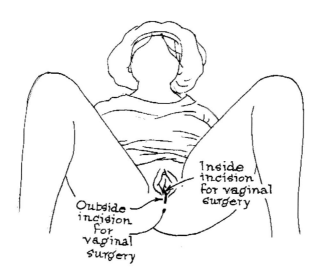

Typically, the patient will stay in the hospital overnight (sometimes two nights) and will completely recover within five to six weeks of surgery. The downside to having vaginal surgery is that the vaginal vault procedure can be difficult to perform and must be done by a highly trained surgeon. The vaginal procedures are also less resilient over long periods of time; they have a higher prolapse recurrence rate. Since a prolapse can come back again, it is possible to have vaginal surgery for prolapse at age 50 and require another surgery by age 70, while A-SCP is likely to be effective for longer periods of time. However, patients usually require a two-or three-day hospital stay for the latter. And having surgery through your belly usually adds one to two additional weeks to your recovery time.

To overcome the higher recurrence rates of vaginal surgery and to maintain the minimally invasive nature of vaginal procedures, surgeons have recently augmented the vaginal prolapse repairs by placing one or more pieces of synthetic mesh through the vagina to add extra reinforcement to the repair. Mesh has been used for over 60 years for abdominal hernia repairs and is considered safe. Unfortunately, the interior of the vagina doesn't react the same way as the abdominal wall when it is exposed to mesh. Based on the evidence that we have until now, a synthetic mesh placed into the interior of the vagina (through an incision) may reduce prolapse recurrence rate, but this comes at a price. Sometimes, patients have to return to the operating room in order to treat complications that occur after surgery. Problems can occur either because of the synthetic mesh and the body's reaction to it, or because of faulty surgical technique. Problems such as erosion of the mesh through the vagina, infection, bleeding, pain, inability to have intercourse, incontinence, recurrence of the prolapse, and fistula (or communication between two organs) can occur. As a result, the FDA issued a warning about the safety of these meshes to would-be patients in October 2008, and this safety warning was strengthened in July 2011. In January 2012, The FDA required additional research (a.k.a. 522 Orders) to address specific safety and effectiveness concerns related to transvaginal mesh for POP. For more details, go to the FDA website: www.fda.gov/medicaldevices/safety/alertsandnotices/ucm262435.htm.

The FDA advisory panel has concluded that both the A-SCP and minimally invasive surgery done for incontinence called midurethral slings (i.e. TVT and TOT), which use a small mesh tape, are both safe and effective in the long term. As discussed above, the jury is still out on prolapse repairs using pieces of synthetic meshes, placed through the interior of vagina (i.e., prolapse repairs done through the vagina using mesh). Routine use of transvaginal mesh is not appropriate. It is our opinion that due to a higher level of FDA scrutiny over this matter and the public's reaction to the FDA statements, it is likely that use of vaginal mesh for prolapse will become less popular in the future. In our practice, when patients ask us for a second opinion, we advise them to be careful not to have any material inserted into their body until there is a minimum of five years of scientific evidence supporting its use. For reasons that are currently not completely understood, synthetic mesh used for hernia repair, for abdominal prolapse repair, and for midurethral slings is safe and effective.

Laparoscopic or Robotic Surgery

Wouldn't it be nice to have a minimally invasive procedure that is effective for a long period of time and doesn't have the complications that we just described? For some patients, the laparoscopic sacrocolpopexy (L-SCP) offers the advantages of the A-SCP and vaginal prolapse surgery without the disadvantages of each. Of course, this surgery requires more skill than performing the A-SCP since it has to be done through four or five keyhole openings in the abdomen. The surgeon inserts small instruments through these tiny keyholes and performs the operation just like an A-SCP. Although the L-SCP does not have as many years of scientific evidence behind it, if the surgical steps are done exactly the same way as the A-SCP, then it should be just as effective. So far the scientific evidence is in favor of the L-SCP. There are few surgeons that can perform the L-SCP without compromising surgical technique. Robotic SCP (R-SCP) allows the surgeon to perform SCP with increased dexterity and accuracy, and can enhance surgical technique.

A Closer Look at Vaginal Surgery

Regardless of which procedure you choose, many doctors will suggest doing several procedures at once since most women have multiple defects and weaknesses in the connective tissues. An anterior repair is used to correct a cystocele (pronounced *SIS-tow-seal)*. This occurs when the tissue that support the bladder (the pubocervical septum) stretches, tears, or detaches from the pelvic floor muscles. After an anterior repair, the bladder will once again sit on top of the hammock, as it once did when you were younger.

Another vaginal approach to fix a protrusion of the rectum into the vagina, called a rectocele (pronounced *REK-tow-seal)*, is by performing a posterior repair. This procedure corrects the rectovaginal septum to restore the connective tissue around the vagina.

Finally, if you're having vaginal surgery, the most important aspect of the prolapse repair, and again, one that requires a properly trained surgeon, is the vaginal vault suspension procedure.

Another way to think about a vaginal vault prolapse is by imagining a sock that has been turned inside out (see drawing of vault prolapse on the next page). A vaginal vault suspension is a procedure used to correct a vaginal vault prolapse (or enterocele) by using sutures to suspend the top of the vagina to one or two of its original ligaments (for example the uterosacral ligaments). A common procedure to fix the vaginal vault is called a uterosacral ligament colposuspension (See Glossary of Operations).

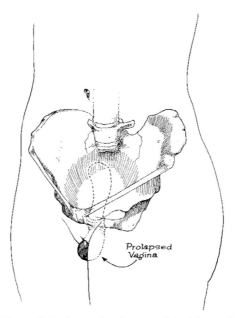

Vaginal Prolapse (sock turned inside out)

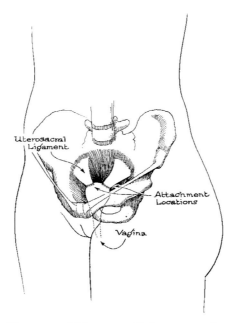

Uterosacral Ligament Colposuspension

By fixing the vaginal vault prolapse, we essentially take the sock that was turned inside out, and we return the sock to its normal shape. A normal-looking sock is just like a normal-looking vagina (see figure on previous page).

Finally, there is one last method to skin the cat so to speak. In an elderly woman who is not sexually active, the sock can be surgically returned to its normal shape and the vaginal opening almost completely shut—this is called colpectomy and colpocleisis. (See "Glossary of *Down There* Operations" at the end of the book). This procedure avoids the need for a hysterectomy. It also has the advantages of being faster (less than one hour) and having minimal risk since it can be done under local anesthesia with sedation. Generally, patients are very satisfied with the outcome after this type of surgery. We will discuss this type of vaginal surgery in one of the cases below.

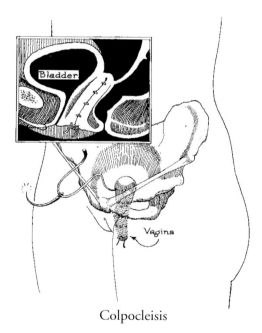

Colpocleisis

In the end, surgery is the only definitive way to fix POP. Just as there are many ways to skin a cat, there are just as many techniques to fix prolapse. The decision on the type of surgical repair is based on age, severity and type of prolapse, sexual activity, level of activity, and willingness to accept or reject the risks associated with one method over another. Let's discuss four patients who presented to us with prolapse and how we individualized their treatments by taking into account their unique circumstances.

Stacy is a 40-year-old advertising executive with red hair and pale skin. She is the mother of two children, and because of heavy vaginal bleeding, had a vaginal hysterectomy five years ago, though her ovaries were not removed. She is very active, runs daily, and is a member of the community tennis association. She also has a Labrador retriever and walks her dog around the neighborhood once a day. She and her husband enjoy an active sex life, but over the last year, she has developed pain during intercourse, and her husband has noticed that he bumps into something during sex. She feels like there's something in the way. He is afraid that he is causing her pain and, as a result, is becoming less enthusiastic about sex. Her prolapse symptoms include a large bulge from her vagina and occasional low back pain that is very uncomfortable and disruptive to her active lifestyle. She also goes to the bathroom numerous times throughout the day even though she doesn't drink excessive amounts of fluid.

For Stacy, we recommended the sacrocolpopexy because she is young and has at least another 35 years of life expectancy. She needs an operation that is going to be strong and last her a very long time. Moreover, because she wants to minimize pain, hospital stay, and downtime after surgery, we recommended a robotic-assisted laparoscopic sacrocolpopexy (R-SCP).

In another case, Marla, a 74-year-old mother of four and grandmother of 10, came to us complaining of a vaginal bulge, which she could feel with her fingers. She often had trouble emptying her bladder and often had to lean forward in order to urinate. She had been worried, wondering if the bulge is related to her difficulty peeing. She is sexually active, although she admits that it has been more difficult to do so because of the prolapse. Her daily activities include watching television, reading, taking a 15-minute walk, cooking, and keeping her house tidy.

After discussing with her the risks, benefits, and alternatives to surgery, she elected to undergo attachment of the top of the vagina to the uterosacral ligaments using sutures and then a suture repair of the front (pubocervical septum) and back (rectovaginal septum) of the vagina (see Glossary of *Down There* Operations); this is entirely a vaginal operation with no incisions on the belly. Marla is not as active as Stacy. Marla wants to remain sexually active and wants an effective surgery that can be accomplished in a minimally invasive fashion.

In another case, Edna, who is an 87-year-old woman, was brought in to see us by her daughter, complaining of vaginal discomfort. When examined, she had a protrusion from her vagina the size of a newborn baby's head! Edna is a very pleasant lady who has multiple medical problems (such as diabetes, high blood pressure, and osteoporosis), but all these are well controlled. She has been living in a retirement home for the last five years. She moved there about the time when her husband passed away. She told us that she has not been sexually active for more than 10 years and is absolutely not interested in that anymore even if she met someone. She spends most of her day participating in activities and classes that are offered. Over the last 30 years or so, her daughter has taken her to all of her medical appointments and has made sure that her mother sees a doctor regularly. She has had normal Pap smears and never complained of any vaginal spotting of blood after menopause. In the past, she tried using different pessaries, but they either didn't work for her—as she said, they "just did not agree with" her.

After talking to Edna about the risks, benefits, and alternatives to surgery, we recommended a fast one-hour procedure (called colpocleisis) with minimal surgical risk and blood loss, which is important for the elderly or those with medical problems. It also offers a very short recovery period. Although a hysterectomy is *not* performed, the vagina is extremely tightened and shortened (i.e. no possibility for intercourse in the future, though sexual intimacy is still possible!). As we have mentioned before, during this operation, the prolapse is surgically placed back inside the vagina, and the vaginal opening is narrowed. No openings or cuts are made in the belly. This operation works extremely well for patients who make an informed decision and who are good candidates. Since a hysterectomy is not done, your doctor will want to make sure that you are not at risk for cervical or endometrial cancers. The entire operation can be done under local anesthetic and sedation without being completely put to sleep (general anesthesia), and it can be completed in approximately one hour. Edna chose to have this operation because sexual activity is not an issue for her. She and her daughter wanted to minimize the amount of time that Edna spends in the operating room and in the hospital (one night). She is hoping to get back to her retirement home as soon as possible so she doesn't miss out on the activities and gossip.

Sharon's case is different. The 55-year-old married, mother of one came to see us with a general feeling that something was not right down there. On our examination, she had a severe uterine prolapse, cystocele, and rectocele. She had seen several doctors in her city and was told by all of them that she needs to have a hysterectomy in order to have her prolapse fixed. She told us that she doesn't believe in a hysterectomy, and she wants to keep all the organs that she was born with. She is a firm believer in naturopathic medicine and wants as little disrupted as possible to fix her prolapse.

Sharon said, "If I don't have cancer in my uterus, then why should I remove it?"

We obtained her medical records, which show that she is healthy and she has had normal Pap smears throughout her lifetime. She has not had any spotting of blood through her vagina since menopause.

After discussing the risks and alternatives, she chose to have a combined robotic assisted attachment of her uterus to her sacrum and a vaginal repair of her prolapse (see Glossary of *Down There* Operations under "Sacrocolpo-cervicohysteropexy"). As a result, she was able to retain her uterus. This operation is accomplished by two minimally invasive routes. After a one-night stay in the hospital and four weeks of recovering, Sharon felt normal again. She went back to her doctors and told them that her prolapse was no longer there, and they were stunned!

Now that we have discussed all the ins and outs of prolapse, let's go back to our original patient. Melissa had a severe prolapse and was worried that the looseness inside her vagina was getting in the way of her and her husband's sexual enjoyment, and so began to withdraw from any sexual encounters. And though she has not gone through menopause yet, her periods have been becoming irregular. She wouldn't mind not having periods anymore, especially since she may not go through menopause for several more years. She also tells us that she has been married for over 30 years and is in a stable monogamous relationship. She has only been with one other man in her entire life.

Her Pap smears have always been normal; so after discussing the risks, benefits, and alternatives to surgery, she chose to have robotic partial hysterectomy with attachment of her vagina and cervix to the sacrum, as well as repair of the opening of the vagina (see Glossary of *Down There* Operations for more detail). What does all this mean? If having surgery was like choosing a dish at a gourmet restaurant, then this operation is considered à la carte! First of all, the entire operation is done in a minimally invasive fashion (laparoscopic) in order to reduce down time. The robotic component is added not only to increase accuracy and precision but also to improve the surgeon's dexterity and visualization. By doing a partial hysterectomy (a.k.a. supracervical hysterectomy), the patient can keep her cervix, which is desired by some women for their own personal reasons even though there is no evidence that keeping the cervix improves sexual function. At the same time, we removed her uterus, which is responsible for her undesired periods. The partial hysterectomy is controversial because doctors who are opposed to this surgery state that a woman will continue to have risk for cervical cancer since her cervix was not removed. Their other concern is that if cancer does develop in the future and the patient is a surgical candidate, the surgery will be more risky and difficult to perform. See Chapter Ten for an explanation of why if you're having your uterus removed, a partial hysterectomy is beneficial when performed at the same time as a L-SCP or a R-SCP.

We also did counsel Melissa that she will need to have regular pelvic examinations and Pap smears since she wants to keep her cervix. The partial hysterectomy is described in Chapter Ten. The attachment of the vagina and cervix to the sacrum is performed by suturing a piece of mesh to all of these structures (see Glossary of *Down There* Operations). Then the opening of the vagina is reduced to normal. This will make her tighter, and both she and her husband will have more sexual enjoyment. And of course, her ovaries were not removed, and thus, she can continue to benefit from the natural hormones that help keep her young and vibrant. Voilá! Magnifique!

After the above surgery, Melissa stayed in the hospital overnight and recovered almost completely in about four weeks. We have seen her back again several times, but at two months after surgery, both she and her husband were extremely happy with the results. Their sex life has improved dramatically! She has recommended us to all of her friends.

The Bottom Line

Prolapse doesn't mean you have to stop having a meaningful and enjoyable lifestyle. It is a common condition, and nearly everyone can be helped. So if you feel or see a bulge down there, see your doctor and get 'er done!

Chapter Four

When It Really Hurts Down There:
Painful Bladder Syndrome

Karen goes to the restroom to urinate more than 20 times a day. As her bladder fills with urine, she experiences pain and the severe urge to urinate. She is up every hour and wakes up exhausted each morning. She knows the location of every restroom within five miles of her home. She has seen several doctors and been treated with antibiotics as if she had a urinary tract infection. The antibiotics usually do not resolve her pain. She also has severe pain with sexual intimacy, which is an added stress to her marriage. She is depressed and is taking multiple medications, including antidepressants. She is a prisoner of her pelvis—located "down there."

Although it's not a malignant or infectious condition, interstitial cystitis (pronounced *in-tur-STISH-ul sis-TI-tis*) / painful bladder syndrome (IC/PBS) can be as disabling and sometimes difficult to manage. Many women undergo ineffective gynecologic surgery in a desperate attempt to subdue their pain.

Knowing When You Have Interstitial Cystitis

IC is a common, but poorly understood, condition that affects one million Americans, mostly women; neither cause nor cure is known. Fortunately, if the condition is identified, help is available, and nearly everyone who suffers from IC can be helped. IC is also called painful bladder syndrome and sometimes even confused with pelvic pain syndrome because of the nature of its symptoms. Classically, women with IC/PBS complain of bladder pain, urgency of urination, frequency of urination, getting up at night to urinate, and burning with urination. Because these women are going to the bathroom so frequently, they will often void only small volumes of urine. Bladder emptying may provide some short-term relief from symptoms, but women with IC/PBS are often miserable, and some are depressed. IC/PBS definitely decreases the quality of life.

Why does it happen?

Your bladder is shaped like a balloon and is located in the pelvis. It has the ability to expand and contract just like a balloon. It has two tubes, ureters that transport urine that is made in the kidneys to bladder where it is stored. There is another small tube, the urethra, that allows the urine to leave the bladder into the toilet when the woman has the desire to urinate. Normally the bladder is able to expand and hold fluid or urine without any discomfort. However, in patients with IC/PBS, the expansion stretches the muscles, which, in turn, irritates the nerves that supply the bladder and causes severe pain. As a result, women with IC/PBS have intense pain as the bladder expands, which also makes them feel that they always have to go to the bathroom. Most women find that the pain in the pelvis will subside after they urinate. In severe cases, even after urinating, the pain will persist.

The best explanation we have today of the cause of IC/PBS is that there is a defect in the lining of the bladder that enables a toxic chemical in the urine to penetrate and irritate the muscles and the nerves that supply the bladder, resulting in the urge to urinate. As the lining becomes more leaky, fibrosis or scar tissue forms in the muscles of the bladder, which decreases the capacity of the bladder to expand when fluid is added to the bladder from the kidneys. This situation then causes women to have a smaller bladder capacity and have to urinate more frequently.

In addition to the urinating symptoms, women with IC/PBS have painful intercourse. Since the bladder is located at the top of the vagina, anything inserted into the vagina—such as a penis, tampon, finger, or a vibrating device—will press against the top of the vagina and irritate the bladder, causing severe pain. Women with IC/PBS will avoid sexual intimacy, which significantly impacts their relationship with their partner.

Holly had severe pain with sexual intimacy. She tried to acclimate herself by using a very small vibrator, but even the smallest device or toy resulted in excruciating pain. In addition, sitting for prolonged periods of time caused her to experience pain and discomfort. She also had urinary frequency and urgency. She felt that she was a prisoner of the toilet. She was examined by nearly a half dozen primary care doctors and gynecologists. She was treated with multiple courses of antibiotics even though she never had a documented urinary tract infection. She was treated with cold compresses and antidepressants without improvement. She was provided with a diagnosis of vulvodynia and told that very little could be done for her, which made her depression even worse. We saw Holly and noted that she had some relief after she urinated, and we suspected that she had IC. She had cystoscopy and hydrodistension, or distension of the bladder with sterile water. Subsequently, the medication, DMSO (dimethyl sulfoxide), was placed in the bladder and she was treated with Elavil and Elmiron (pentosan polysulfate). After several months, she noted moderate improvement in her pain and discomfort. She was also able to engage in sexual intimacy with her husband, and her marriage was saved.

Now you can see why women with IC/PBS are prisoners of their bladders. They know the location of every toilet within miles of their home or their work. It is difficult for women with IC/PBS to be productive in the workplace, as they have to go to the bathroom so frequently. Any interruption of work, be it taking a phone call, answering a text message, or dealing with an e-mail, results in a loss of focus. When a woman with IC/PBS has to leave the workplace two to three times an hour, it is not hard to imagine that there is a loss of focus and a loss of productivity. It is quite common for many women with IC to consult with five or even more doctors before the diagnosis is made. And some are wrongly diagnosed and given prescriptions of antibiotics, which are ineffective since there is no bacteria or evidence of infection causing the problem.

Many women are told that it is "in their head" and given anti-anxiety medications, but these alone are not going to treat the problem. Women become depressed and despondent because of the incapacitating bladder condition down there and will often be sent to a counselor or psychiatrist. This too will not completely solve the problem. It is not hard to understand why women with IC/PBS are miserable as this incapacitating condition can end-up controlling every waking moment of a woman's life.

Diagnosis of IC/PBS Is Tricky

To most physicians, IC/PBS appears to be a very common condition that is often underdiagnosed or improperly diagnosed. The number of people affected is somewhat controversial but estimates in the United States are around 70 out of every 100,000, and the condition is most common in women over age 40. Your doctor must have an awareness of the disease and its symptoms in order to make the diagnosis. We both have seen patients who come to the office for an appointment or are self-referred, and they have made the diagnosis themselves from their own research on the Internet.

Unfortunately, unlike the garden-variety urinary tract infection (discussed in Chapter Five), which can be diagnosed with a simple urine test that can be done in the doctor's office, there is no test or tests that can be performed that will conclude that a woman has IC/PBS. Consequently, IC is often considered a diagnosis of exclusion—that is, other causes of pelvic pain and urinary symptoms must be ruled out first, and if none of those conditions are present, then a diagnosis of IC/PBS is made.

If your doctor suspects you have IC/PBS, he/she must rule out other treatable conditions before considering a diagnosis of IC/PBS. The most common of these diseases are urinary tract infections and endometriosis. Bladder cancer is also a cause of pelvic pain (see Chapter Five). (Please do keep in mind that IC/PBS is not associated with any increased risk of developing cancer.)

The Diagnosis of IC/PBS Is Based On:

- Presence of pain related to the bladder, usually accompanied by frequency and urgency of urination;
- Absence of other diseases that could cause the symptoms; and
- Dyspareunia or painful intercourse.

Diagnostic tests that help rule out other diseases include urinalysis, urine culture, cystoscopy, biopsy of the bladder wall and urethra, and distention of the bladder under anesthesia.

If your doctor suspects that you may have IC/PBS, he/she may perform a cystoscopic examination in order to rule out bladder cancer.

During cystoscopy, the doctor uses a cystoscope—an instrument made of a small hollow tube about the diameter of a drinking straw with several lenses and a light—to see inside the bladder and urethra. The doctor might also distend or stretch the bladder to its capacity by filling it with a liquid, such as sterile water or saline, which is a salt solution. Because bladder distention is painful for people with IC/PBS, they must be given some form of anesthesia for the procedure. The classic finding at the time of cystoscopy is the presence of small ulcers of the lining of the bladder and bleeding under the bladder lining (referred to as petechiae). If a bladder biopsy is performed, scarring or fibrosis and an accumulation of mast cells, which are part of the immune system and responsible for the release of histamine that causes the inflammation and pain, will be found under the bladder lining when the tissue is examined under the microscope.

While you are under anesthesia, your doctor will measure the capacity of the bladder, or how much the bladder will hold. This is usually not done when the patient is awake as it is too painful. If the bladder capacity is less than 350 cc or about 12 oz., this is highly suggestive of IC/PBS if the woman has the symptoms of bladder pain, frequency, and urgency of urination, and the urine exam is negative for infection or blood. The small bladder capacity is a consequence of scarring of the bladder, making it difficult to hold urine, and results in the frequency of urination and the pain associated with filling of the bladder with urine.

Unfortunately, no other laboratory or imaging studies aid in diagnosis. After these evaluations are completed, confirmation of the diagnosis depends on the cystoscopic findings. Hydrodistention of the bladder is often performed during cystoscopy, while the patient is under the anesthesia. Hydrodistention consists of filling the bladder with saline or a salt solution or sterile water beyond its normal capacity. Pinpoint hemorrhages or fissures with bleeding may appear after the distention. Although hydrodistention of the bladder is used in diagnosis of IC, it also provides symptomatic relief to some women, for reasons that are not understood.

Getting the Right Treatment for Your Pain Down There

Doctors have tried many methods of providing relief from symptoms of IC. However, no standard or universally accepted treatment has been found that reliably and invariably resolves this debilitating condition.

Roberta has mild IC/PBS and had exacerbations when she was sleep deprived and under stress. She was able to relieve the symptoms with cold compresses applied to the exterior of her vagina and lower abdomen. She also used an over-the-counter medication, quercitin, which also seemed to alleviate her symptoms.

Marilyn had daily symptoms and had difficulty holding a job because she was always in the restroom. She had seen several primary care doctors, several gynecologists, and a urologist before she was diagnosed with IC/PBS. She finally achieved relief following a bladder hydrodistension, the use of oral medication, heparin placed in her bladder, and 10 mg of Elavil every evening.

Olivia, age 47, was almost totally incapacitated with her IC/PBS. Her problem took years to diagnose and also resulted in the dissolution of her marriage of 25 years. Her frequency was noted at 45 times a day and 15 to 20 times a night. Her bladder capacity was less than 3 oz. or 90 cc. She had an Interstim device inserted, which was an attempt to modulate her severe frequency and urgency, without success. Finally, she had her bladder removed and, with psychotherapy, was slowly able to put her life back in order.

Because the cause of IC is unknown, doctors alternate between oral medications, such as pentosan polysulfate (Elmiron, the only medicine that is FDA approved). Elmiron, which is a blood thinner or anticoagulant, is a fairly new drug treatment for IC/PBS that works by coating the inner lining of the bladder that becomes damaged by the disease and helps to restore the inner lining toward normal.

Many women with IC/PBS find that if they are going to see any positive effects with Elmiron, it takes between three to six months, and some opt to keep trying for as long a year. A decrease in pain is often one of the first reported positive effects, with fewer frequency and urgency symptoms following. It appears that about 35 to 40 percent of women with IC/PBS who take Elmiron notice marked improvement.

Elmiron is a very safe drug, and only a few women with IC/PBS experience side effects such as diarrhea or nausea. An uncommon side effect is hair loss, which occurs in about 3 percent of the women who use Elmiron. Fortunately, the hair loss is temporary, and the hair will grow back once the medication is discontinued.

The tricyclic antidepressant amitriptyline may help reduce pain, increase bladder capacity, and decrease frequency and nocturia or night-time voiding. Some women may not be able to tolerate amitriptyline because it may make them tired during the day. One solution is to take the medication in the evening before going to sleep, and this may help reduce day-time lethargy. In women with severe pain, narcotic analgesics such as acetaminophen (Tylenol) with codeine or longer-acting narcotics may occasionally be necessary.

Use of hydroxyzine (Atarax), an antihistamine, is also effective especially if the biopsy of the bladder shows an excess of mast cells, which release histamine and is responsible for the pain in the bladder.

Another oral medication that has been effective for treating IC\PBS is cimetidine (Tagamet), which is an over-the-counter drug used to treat peptic ulcer disease. The dosage is 300 mg twice a day. The drug is well tolerated and has few side effects. How cimetidine works in the treatment of IC/PBS has not been fully worked out.

Other oral medications include anticholinergic drugs, such as Ditropan, Detrol, Vesicare, Toviaz, Enablex, and Sanctura, which are used to decrease bladder spasms. There are bladder analgesics such as Pyridium, which turns the urine orange but can relieve the pain associated with urination. Other medications that may reduce the symptoms of IC include sedatives for those women who have trouble getting and staying asleep.

Medications that Soothe the Pain Down There

You can also instill liquid medication into the bladder through a temporary catheter that is inserted through the urethra into the bladder. The medication remains in the bladder for as long as possible (ideally 30 minutes to one hour); then a woman empties the remainder of the medication when she goes to the bathroom. This treatment option has very few side effects since so little of the medication is absorbed from the bladder and is usually not very painful or even uncomfortable.

Many medications have been instilled into the bladder through a small tube or catheter in an attempt to relieve symptoms. Today, the most commonly used medication that is instilled in the bladder is dimethyl sulfoxide (DMSO) or RIMSO. DMSO is approved by the FDA for the treatment of IC/PBS. Although DMSO is an anti-inflammatory agent, it seems to have some pain-relieving properties as well. As is true of other therapies for IC, there is no way to predict which women will respond to DMSO.

DMSO treatment regimens vary and have included instillation weekly for six weeks; and especially in patients who do respond, a *booster* dose is given every month. There is no uniformity of choice regarding treatment schedules. Most likely, each doctor uses a slightly different approach; as yet, there is no right way to use DMSO. It is probably safe to say that if a woman with IC/PBS does not experience relief within a few treatments, further instillation of DMSO is unlikely to be effective. The most common side effect of DMSO is a complaint of a garlic-like taste and odor after instillation. Most women will use a peppermint candy after the treatment and don't notice the taste.

Following the initial course of treatment, some patients achieve long-term remission, but most relapse eventually. Additional treatment schedules for those who relapse vary but usually consist of instillation every four to six weeks. There are some women who learn how to insert the small catheter and instill the DMSO in the privacy of their homes and can use the treatment whenever symptoms occur. Sometimes, dimethyl sulfoxide is combined with heparin, cortico steroids, bicarbonate, and a local anesthetic (xylocaine) as a bladder treatment. If DMSO does not relieve your symptoms, your doctor may try heparin combined with local anesthetic. This is successful in some patients who do not respond to DMSO.

Botox Is Not Just for Wrinkles

Botox—which has been used for years to plump up the skin and wipe away those wrinkles around the eyes, mouth, and forehead—now has a role in the treatment of IC/PBS. Recently, researchers have been investigating its use for injection into the bladder muscle to reduce bladder spasms in patients with IC/PBS who have not responded to oral medication or bladder instillations.

Botox is made from the botulinum toxin, modified and utilized in FDA-approved procedures such as for the treatment of wrinkles. By injecting Botox into a woman's bladder, the nerves are essentially put to sleep, calming their harmful influence on the bladder. Unfortunately, Botox does not cure the problem and must be repeated every three to 12 months.

For a patient with IC/PBS, the procedure is usually done in the operating room where a very tiny needle is inserted through a cystoscope, and the bladder muscle is injected at multiple locations with Botox. Improvement is seen within a few days; and if there is improvement, it will last from four to six months, and then the procedure can be repeated.

Most insurance companies do not authorize or reimburse patients for the use of Botox for IC/PBS. It is, however, approved for urinary symptoms in patients with multiple sclerosis and neurogenic bladder overactivity.

Helping Your IC/PBS Through Diet

Many women with the IC/PBS find that eliminating or reducing their intake of potential bladder irritants may help to relieve their discomfort. The most irritating foods can be summarized as the four Cs:

- Carbonated beverages
- Caffeine in all forms (including chocolate);
- Citrus fruits and juices; and
- Vitamin C (and foods containing it and potassium).

If you find that your bladder is irritated by these things, you may also wish to avoid related foods such as tomatoes, pickled foods, alcohol, and spices. Artificial sweeteners may aggravate symptoms in some women as well. If you think certain foods make you feel worse, try eliminating them from your diet. Reintroduce them one at a time to determine which, if any, affect your signs and symptoms.

Most women can identify the culprits by conducting a simple elimination diet. We suggest that you stop eating all the foods on the bladder irritant list shown at the end of the chapter. We recommend that you adhere to this elimination diet for two weeks. If the bladder symptoms improve, then you can be sure that one or several of the foods or liquids was irritating your bladder. Then begin by eating just one food from the bladder irritant list. If you don't develop any symptoms of pelvic pain or increase in urinary urgency or frequency within 24 hours, then you can be reasonably certain that this is not one of the foods or fluids that is affecting your IC/PBS. You can then add one new food or liquid each day until you have identified the offending foods that are making you so miserable. Additional treatments for IC involve maintaining healthy lifestyle habits, particularly for the bladder. This means getting optimal amounts of water, 60 ounces a day or more. The bladder should be emptied regularly throughout the day and always after intercourse. Again, improving the diet seems to play a significant role in decreasing symptoms. We always question toxin exposure with IC sufferers as we both have had a few patients who live near areas with higher levels of various toxins and removal from the toxins reduced their symptoms of IC. Drinking filtered water, such as with reverse osmosis filtration, is also recommended.

Coping with Your IC/PBS

There is probably no problem in the pelvis that requires a more sympathetic family and significant other. Emotional support is very important in coping with ongoing pain and the necessity of going to the restroom so frequently. Family and friends can often supply the support. However, you are not alone, and there are excellent support groups that meet on a regular basis, and the Internet also has support groups of individuals with IC/PBS, and they are usually very helpful. (See resources at the end of the chapter for support groups near you.)

Here are some tips to remember:

- Find a healthcare team that is sympathetic and helpful.
- Understand that your healthcare team does not know all the answers and may be as frustrated as you are.
- Stay in touch with family and friends. Don't become isolated.
- Involve your family in treatment decisions.
- Remember that IC is only one part of your life. Don't allow it to become all of your life.
- Talk to others about their experiences and ways of coping.
- Wear loose clothing. Avoid belts or clothes that put pressure on your abdomen.
- Reduce stress. Try methods such as visualization and biofeedback, and low-impact exercise. (See Chapter Thirteen.)
- Stop smoking, as the active ingredient in tobacco, nicotine, may worsen any painful condition, and smoking is harmful to the bladder.
- Try pelvic floor physiotherapy. See a physical therapist trained in pelvic floor disorders, or a women's clinical specialist. The physiotherapist will gently stretch and release the pelvic floor muscles and this may reduce muscle spasms and pain. Pelvic

floor physiotherapists sometimes combine this technique with biofeedback.

When All Else Fails: Surgery

By far, most women with IC/PBS can be helped with medications, drugs placed in the bladder, and hydrodistension. However, there are a few unfortunate women, such as Holly, for whom nothing seems to help. They have tried all of the conservative approaches and have seen multiple physicians and experts who treat IC/PBS, and yet the women remain miserable and incapacitated by the disease. In these few women, a surgical option may be the only solution.

Attempts have been made to sever the nerves to the bladder that appear to be associated with the pain and discomfort. Occasionally, some women will have a part or even all the bladder removed. For those women with IC/PBS who have a very small bladder that holds only a small volume of urine, they may have their bladder capacity augmented by attaching a piece of intestine to the bladder in order to increase the bladder capacity.

Nerve Stimulation

If you have tried diet changes, exercise, and medicines and nothing seems to help, you may wish to think about nerve stimulation. This treatment sends mild electrical pulses to the nerves that control the bladder.

At first, you may try a system that sends the pulses through electrodes placed on your skin. If this therapy works for you, you may consider having a device put in your body. The device delivers small pulses of electricity to the nerves around the bladder.

For some patients, nerve stimulation relieves bladder pain as well as urinary frequency and urgency. For others, the treatment relieves frequency and urgency but not pain. For still other patients, it does not work.

The treatment consists of electrical pulses, which block the pain signals carried in the nerves. If your brain doesn't receive the nerve signal, you don't feel the pain. Mild electrical pulses can be used to stimulate the nerves to the bladder—either through the skin or with an implanted device. The method of delivering impulses through the skin is called transcutaneous electrical nerve stimulation (TENS). With TENS, mild electric pulses enter the body for minutes to hours, two or more times a day either through wires placed on the lower back or just above the pubic area—between the navel and the pubic hair—or through special devices inserted into the vagina. The electrical pulses may increase blood flow to the bladder, strengthen pelvic muscles that help control the bladder, or trigger the release of substances that block pain.

TENS is relatively inexpensive and allows people with IC/PBS to take an active part in treatment. Within some guidelines, the patient decides when, how long, and at what intensity TENS will be used. It has been most helpful in relieving pain and decreasing frequency of urination. Smokers do not respond as well as nonsmokers. If TENS is going to help, improvement is usually apparent in three to four months.

You may also consider having a device, InterStim™, implanted underneath your skin in the buttocks area so that it can deliver regular impulses to the sacral nerves which go to your pelvis. A wire is placed next to the tailbone and attached to a permanent stimulator under the skin. The FDA has approved this device to treat IC/PBS when other treatments have not worked. Chapter 2 has more information about InterStim.

For the Most Difficult Cases

For those women who have severe scarring of the bladder and who are unable to hold even a modest amount of fluid, they can be offered a bladder augmentation, which makes the bladder larger. In most of these procedures, scarred, ulcerated, and inflamed sections of the bladder are removed, leaving only the base of the bladder and healthy tissue. A piece of the colon (large intestine) is then removed, reshaped, and attached to what remains of the bladder. After the incisions heal, you may have to urinate less often. The effect on pain varies greatly; IC can sometimes affect the segment of colon used to enlarge the bladder.

The last-straw solution is to totally remove the bladder, called a cystectomy. Fortunately, it is rarely used. Once the bladder has been removed, different methods can be used to reroute the urine. In most cases, ureters are attached to a piece of colon that opens onto the skin of the abdomen. This procedure is called a urostomy, and the opening is called a stoma. Urine empties through the stoma into a bag outside the body.

So What Happened to Our Patient Karen?

She had a cystoscopy, bladder hydrodistension, and a bladder biopsy, which confirmed the diagnosis of IC/PBS. She was placed on Elmiron and had a six-week course of bladder instillations with DMSO. She has had marked improvement in her symptoms of frequency and urgency. She is also able to engage in sexual intimacy without pain and discomfort. Just like in the fairy tales, she and her husband are living happily ever after!

Our advice: Start with the simplest self-care strategies, such as wearing loose clothing and limiting soda, caffeine, citrus fruits and juices. Wait a reasonable amount of time to see if these measures help, and keep the trying new ones, as long as they don't disrupt your life even more than IC already has. Perhaps most important, find a compassionate physician who is concerned about your quality of life as well as your condition and will work with you to help alleviate your frequency, urgency, and bladder pain.

Also, you might benefit from joining a support group. Such a group can provide both sympathetic listening and useful information. For a list of interstitial cystitis support groups throughout the United States or for information on how to start a group in your area, contact the Interstitial Cystitis Association on the Web.

The Bottom Line

IC is fairly common in primary care practices and very common in urology practices. Still, it is probably underdiagnosed. Because symptoms can be confusing, patients are sometimes thought to have psychogenic problems or are treated repeatedly with antibiotics, despite the absence of evidence of bacterial infection. The key to correct diagnosis is awareness of the condition and its characteristics. In women who have symptoms that resemble routine cystitis but normal results on urinalysis, interstitial cystitis should be considered as the working diagnosis.

Many doctors do not talk about achieving a cure when dealing with IC, but certainly long-term remission of symptoms is accomplished in many patients because of (or possibly in spite of) various therapies. All therapies for IC/PBS are truly a trial-and-error undertaking, but any method that is safe and relieves symptoms will be well received by the women who suffer from IC/PBS. We suggest you look for a doctor who is knowledgeable about IC/PBS, is a good listener, is caring, and has compassion for those who suffer from this condition.

For More Information
American Urological Association Foundation, 1000 Corporate Boulevard, Linthicum, MD 21090; Phone: 1-866-RING-AUA (1-866-746-4282) or 410-689-3700; Fax: 410-689-3800; E-mail: patienteducation@auafoundation.org; Internet: www. auafoundation.org www.UrologyHealth.org.

Interstitial Cystitis Association, 100 Park Avenue, Suite 108A, Rockville, MD 20850; Phone: 1-800-HELP-ICA (1-800-435-7422) or 301-610-5300; Fax: 301-610-5308; E-mail: ICAmail@ichelp.org; Internet: www.ichelp.org.

National Association For Continence (NAFC) PO Box 1019 Charleston, SC 29402-1019 Phone: 1-800-BLADDER (1-843-377-0900) Internet: www.nafc.org

Chapter Five

When What's Going on Down There Is Not "All In Your Head": Chronic Pelvic Pain

Have you been suffering with pain in your pelvis but have been told that "it's all in your head"? Have you seen numerous doctors and had countless tests that have always turned up normal? Have you been told you have endometriosis or depression but none were proven to be your cause of pelvic pain? Did a doctor ever ask you if you have been sexually abused after you told him/her you have pelvic pain? If you answered yes to any of the above questions, then you may be suffering from a condition known as chronic pelvic pain (CPP).

Chronic pelvic pain is defined as pain below the level of the belly button that has been present for at least six months, but is not cyclic, meaning every month it doesn't go away at a certain part of your menstrual cycle and then return at another part of your cycle. CPP impacts your ability or desire to participate in your regular activities, affects your work, and makes life in general miserable. Because the pain is so chronic (usually nonstop), it can cause havoc in your relationships, trigger depression, and if left untreated, often result in a hysterectomy, often unnecessarily. Indeed, CPP is the single most common reason doctors perform hysterectomies.

As Carolyn, age 53, described, "When my pelvic pain first started five years ago, it felt like aching in my bladder and burning around my vagina. There has always been a constant ache inside my pelvis, but after sex, it flares up and becomes throbbing. I can literally feel my pulse in my vagina. Sometimes, the pain spreads to the areas surrounding my vagina and radiates down my legs. Because of my pelvic pain, I don't enjoy any of the activities that I used to relish. And because sex is so painful, I don't enjoy it anymore. I've stopped having sex with my partner altogether."

And yet despite these life-altering repercussions, more than 15 percent of American women suffer from CPP at one time in their lives. But even more startling, the majority of these women don't seek care from a doctor or other healthcare provider.

Getting to the Root of the Problem

Many conditions can cause pelvic pain (see Table 1), but the challenge is determining which is the accurate cause of the pain. To make matters more frustrating, there is usually more than one cause of the pain. We have both seen patients who have had all the tests that have turned up normal, and no diagnosis was made. Is their pain real? Of course it is. For these women, the condition(s), which started their pain, may have disappeared or have been treated along the way while they sought therapy from various doctors, but now their brain still believes that something painful is happening in the pelvis. This centralization of pain is now the reason for their continued CPP. A somewhat analogous phenomenon happens in people who have had one of their limbs amputated. Many amputees experience painful sensations even though the limb no longer exists.

The long list of conditions that can potentially cause CPP are divided into the following categories:

- Gynecologic (female reproductive organs);
- Gastrointestinal (bowels, rectum, etc.);
- Urologic (bladder, urethra, etc.);
- Musculoskeletal and neurologic (connective tissues, muscles of the abdominal wall and pelvic floor, posture, and nerve compression or injury); and
- Psychiatric (depression, abuse, etc.).

Unless your doctor is a walking encyclopedia, no doctor, by himself/ herself, will have all the expertise to help a patient with pelvic pain. Often a team of healthcare professionals from gynecology, gastroenterology, urology, rheumatology, psychiatry, pain medicine, and physical therapy may be necessary to manage different aspects of care for a person suffering from CPP. This multidisciplinary approach has the highest chance of helping reduce your suffering.

Stopping the Pain

If you and your doctor are certain that one of these conditions is actually causing your pain, then the right treatments have a reasonable chance of succeeding. And obviously, a concerned, thoughtful physician will make every effort to find the reason for your pelvic pain—not only to prevent further injury to your pelvic sensory nerves but also to alleviate the source of discomfort.

A Closer Look at Chronic Pelvic Pain

As physicians, we find CPP a frustrating, challenging conundrum that requires patience and persistence to both diagnose and treat. We know that the pelvic pain is real because we see our patients suffering. It's definitely not in your head. But what's causing it? While we struggle to diagnose the cause of your pelvic pain by putting you through a battery of tests, you continue to endure unnecessarily. We try hard to classify CPP based on the probable origin of pain so that we have some idea of how to help you. We usually classify the origin of CPP as either gynecologic, urologic, gastrointestinal, musculoskeletal, urologic, or psychiatric; these categories helps us sift through the most common diagnoses so that we can come to an accurate assessment as quickly as possible and alleviate the pain of our patients. Let's take a closer look at the conditions that can cause or trigger CPP.

Table 1. **Causes of Chronic Pelvic Pain**

(The most common causes are listed in bold print)

Gynecologic	**Endometriosis** Pelvic and abdominal adhesions Vulvodynia and vulvar vestibulitis Adenomyosis Pelvic congestion syndrome Ovarian remnant syndrome Ovarian cancer Sequelae of pelvic inflammatory disease **Sequelae of prior pelvic surgery** (of cervix, vaginal prolapse repair with mesh, etc.)
Urologic	**Interstitial cystitis** Urethral syndrome Radiation cystitis Bladder cancer Urethral diverticulum Recurrent cystitis and urethritis
Gastrointestinal	**Irritable bowel syndrome** Inflammatory bowel disease (Crohn's and ulcerative colitis) Diverticular disease (diverticulosis and diverticulitis) Constipation Celiac disease Colon cancer Shingles Porphyria Intermittent bowel obstruction Hernia

Musculoskeletal and neurologic	**Myofascial pelvic pain syndrome** Chronic back pain Rectus diastasis Poor posture Fibromyalgia Osteitis pubis Lumbar herniated disc Radiculopathy **Neuropathy** (pudendal nerve injury or entrapment) Degenerative joint disease Orthopedic problems (leg length discrepancy, pelvic obliquity, hip or sacral stress fracture) Pregnancy-and childbirth related (sacroiliac joint dysfunction, pubic symphysis pain)
Psychiatric	**Somatization disorder** Hypochondriasis Depression Bipolar disorder Sexual abuse Substance dependency Sleep disorders

Endometriosis

Women with CPP are given the diagnosis of endometriosis more often than any other diagnosis. One in 10 women from the time she starts menstruation to the time she goes through menopause may develop endometriosis. This condition begins when the lining of the uterus, or the endometrium, starts to travel and grow outside of the uterus. The endometrium can go anywhere in the body, but most often it will go to the ovary and the tissues surrounding the uterus. Once it gets there, the endometrium may cause adhesions between tissues, and over time, it may distort the anatomy of the pelvis. In other words, the freely mobile, slippery, reproductive organs may become encased, twisted, and "frozen" in time and space. It's like Medusa gazing into the pelvis and turning everything into stone! Besides causing scarring, endometriosis can form "chocolate cysts" on top of the ovaries and cause blockage of the bowel. All these effects can lead to symptoms of CPP, which is often worse at some point during menstrual cycle. Endometriosis can also cause cramping, back and leg pain, pain during intercourse, pain during urination, irritable bowel symptoms (described later in this chapter), and infertility. Other symptoms may include headache, anxiety, and chronic weakness. A peculiar feature of this condition is that the amount of endometriosis found at the time of surgery doesn't always correlate with the amount of pain. For example, a woman may have severe endometriosis found during surgery and yet complain of very little pain. Or vice versa, someone may have just a few endometrial implants in her pelvis but have severe pelvic pain.

Additionally, many women are misdiagnosed with endometriosis. The only way to be sure that you actually have endometriosis is by performing a laparoscopy (inserting a narrow camera into the pelvis) and then doing a biopsy of the lesion(s), which is believed to be endometriosis. Only after a pathologist confirms the biopsy can your doctor give you an accurate diagnosis of endometriosis. We often see patients who were labeled with a diagnosis of endometriosis without any confirmation.

If a woman is past her childbearing years or if fertility is not an issue, hormonal treatment can suppress endometriosis. Treatments can include hormones such as oral contraceptives, progesterone, danazol (Danocrine), and leuprolide (Lupron). All these can be taken in the form of a pill, but leuprolide and progesterone are usually injections. None of the treatments are superior to the others. However, a potential benefit of Lupron is that it may work for other conditions causing pelvic pain, including irritable bowel syndrome, pelvic congestion syndrome, and interstitial cystitis. Patients may also take NSAIDS (nonsteroidal anti-inflammatory drugs) and/or pain medication to help relieve their discomfort. Some doctors advocate doing a laparoscopy and use of cautery or laser to destroy the abnormal tissue, or vaporizing the endometriosis. Another option, albeit less popular, for the treatment of pain focused in the center portion of the pelvis is a surgical procedure called presacral neurectomy. A small camera and several small surgical instruments are inserted through several small keyhole incisions on the abdominal wall. The group of nerves which supply the uterus and lay over your sacrum, are then divided. This treatment is not effective for CPP, but may be for central dysmenorrhea, or pain associated with menstruation that is located only in the middle/center of the pelvis. If these treatments don't help, then hysterectomy along with removal of both ovaries is the most definitive treatment of endometriosis. Sometimes, however, even these procedures don't guarantee that your pain will go away completely. Women need to weigh the risks and benefits of removing the ovaries before menopause, as early removal can have adverse consequences, such as loss of certain health benefits and will result in immediate menopause (see Chapter Ten on hysterectomy and Chapter Nine on menopause).

Adenomyosis

Adenomyosis is a condition where the lining of the uterus, called the endometrium, grows inside the muscular wall of the womb. In other words, adenomyosis is like having endometriosis inside the uterus. It causes the uterus to grow in size and feel boggy and heavy. We don't know why it happens, but it can develop after pregnancy and childbirth in some women, but usually occurs between ages 35 and menopause. A woman may have adenomyosis and have absolutely no symptoms; we know this because routinely we examine uteri of patients who do not have pelvic pain and have had hysterectomies, and we find this abnormal tissue in the wall of the uteri. However, some women who have adenomyosis experience painful periods, pelvic pain, and heavy vaginal bleeding. Other than discovering adenomyosis after surgery, the best way to diagnose it before going to the operating room is by doing an MRI of the pelvis.

Medications such as NSAIDs, birth control pills, or other hormones can be successful in treating adenomyosis. In the past, many hysterectomies were done because doctors attributed their patient's symptoms to adenomyosis. Hysterectomy is still an option, but is done less often for this reason.

Adhesions

Normally, the surfaces of the internal organs and tissues are slippery and mobile. When adhesions form, tissues become glued to each other like wet Elmer's glue between two sheets of paper. Adhesions usually form after surgery or because of infections. Most of the time, adhesions don't cause any problems, but in some people, they can cause pain, blockage of the flow of digested food through the intestines, and even infertility. Doctors used to think that adhesions always cause pelvic pain, but we now have a different understanding. In fact, studies show that patients with chronic pelvic pain have the same amount of adhesions as infertility patients who have no pain at all. Additionally, surgical removal of adhesions has not been shown to be beneficial unless the adhesions are thick, dense, and vascular, and they limit movement of the pelvic organs.

Nevertheless, adhesions can be a source of pain in some women. If you and your doctor believe that abdominal and pelvic adhesions may be a source of your CPP, then a diagnostic laparoscopy along with possible lysis of adhesions may be necessary. During this procedure, the surgeon cuts and reduces the adhesions which may be contributing to your pain.

Pelvic congestion syndrome

Pelvic congestion syndrome is a condition where dilated veins in the pelvic and reproductive tract (ovarian veins) cause pelvic pressure and pain. These veins are like varicose veins in the leg. Not all women who have these large veins in their pelvis complain of CPP. However, a patient with CPP who also has varicose veins of the legs, thighs, buttocks, and vagina and who has more pain as the day progresses could have pelvic congestion syndrome.

This condition is thought to begin during pregnancy as hormones and large volume of blood cause the opening of and injury to the valves inside the veins. This enlargement leads to backflow and pooling of blood, which then engorges and stretches the veins in the pelvis. Patients with this condition commonly complain of dull pelvic pain, heaviness, and pressure. These symptoms can often be worse after sexual intercourse, multiple pregnancies, and prolonged standing, and the pain usually subsides when the woman lies down allowing the dilated veins to collapse.

Because an interventional radiologist (a radiology doctor specializing in procedures) looks at veins more often, they are more likely to think about and diagnose you with pelvic congestion than your gynecologist. Despite some gynecologists questioning pelvic congestion syndrome as a real diagnosis, we believe that engorged veins in the pelvis can cause pelvic pain. If a doctor diagnoses you with pelvic congestion syndrome, then you may be a candidate for treatment, which entails embolization of your pelvic veins. This procedure is similar to uterine artery embolization (UAE) except instead of the artery being plugged up, the varicose veins in the pelvis are occluded (see Chapter Ten for complete discussion of UAE). Progestins such as daily medroxyprogesterone acetate may also have some therapeutic benefit in patients with pelvic congestion syndrome. Leuprolide has also been effective in relieving pain in some women. Finally, if you have pelvic congestion syndrome and none of the above treatments has helped your pain, then hysterectomy is probably your best option.

Ovarian remnant syndrome

If a woman has had her ovaries removed but the surgery was difficult because of endometriosis, adhesions, infection, or multiple previous surgeries, there may be a chance that part of an ovary was inadvertently left behind. The remaining ovary can cause problems by forming a cyst and/or being distorted by adhesions and, thus, leading to cyclic pelvic pain. The lump can be about an inch or less in diameter, and the pain is often worsened with intercourse. Sometimes, when the diagnosis is difficult, your doctor may give you hormones to stimulate and enlarge the remaining ovary(ies) so they can be located by ultrasound. If you are diagnosed with ovarian remnant syndrome, you will need to have the remaining piece(s) of the ovary(ies) removed by an experienced gynecologic surgeon.

Vulvodynia

A woman who has chronic pain in the external genitalia, or the vulva, which has no other explanation (in other words, there is no infection or skin condition affecting the vulva) is considered to have vulvodynia..

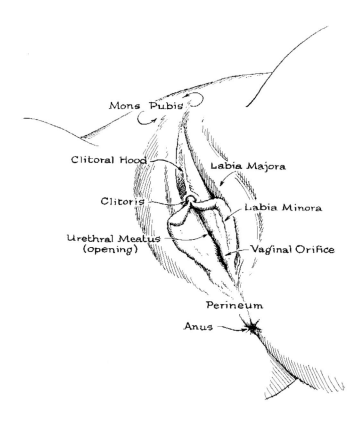

Patients with vulvodynia may also have CPP. Typically, women with vulvodynia experience a stinging, burning, or sharp pain in the opening of the vagina and their labia. As Carolyn said, "Sometimes the pain is constant . . . sometimes it's more intermittent." Often, an activity or pressure on the vulva can trigger pain. Activities that are notorious for starting discomfort and pain include bicycle/horseback riding, inserting a tampon, and sexual intercourse. Vulvodynia can be difficult to distinguish from spasms of muscles surrounding the vagina, or vaginismus.

Unfortunately, there is no universally accepted treatment for vulvodynia. Some women respond well to one therapy such as pelvic floor physical therapy; whereas others may require multiple treatments with modest response. If you think you may have vulvodynia, ask your physician to refer you to a gynecologist who knows how do manage this painful condition. You can also take these steps to help alleviate your discomfort:

1. Wear cotton underwear, skirts, and cotton pads. Try to avoid synthetic fabrics in your underwear or bathing suit. Also, try to avoid wearing tight pants and synthetic pantyhose.

2. Wash down there gently and with cold water only. Avoid using soaps, especially fragrant soaps. Avoid using perfume down there. Avoid laundry detergents that are aromatic.

3. Try a low-oxalate diet. Oxalate salts are by-products of certain types of food, such as spinach, peanuts, soybeans, wheat bran, chocolate, and strawberries. They are excreted in the urine and can form crystals that can irritate the vulva when urine touches it. Foods such as nuts, seeds, berries, carrots, cocoa, and wheat products tend to form high amounts of oxalate salts in your urine and should be avoided. The following is a list of foods that either do not contain or contain very low amounts of oxalate:

No Oxalate

Bacon
Baking soda
Beef
Club soda
Eggs
Fish
Ham
Lamb
Meats
Pork
Port wine
Alcoholic beverage
Poultry
Pumpkin raw
Radishes red
Shellfish
Sherry
Watercress

Very Low Oxalate

Acorn squash
Aloe vera juice
Apple cider vinegar
Apple juice
Apricots fresh
Aspartame
Avocados
Baking powder
Bok choy
Butter
Buttermilk
Cauliflower boiled
Cheddar cheese
Cherries fresh
Chestnuts

Chives
Cilantro
Coconut
Coffee
Coffee (instant)
Corn syrup
Courgette (zucchini)
Cranberry juice
Cream of tartar
Cucumbers
Echinacea
Evaporated cane juice
Gelatin (unflavored)
Ghee
Grapefruit juice
Grapes green
Green beans
Honey
Honeydew
Ketchup
Kohlrabi
Kumquats
Lecithin (soy)
Lemons
Lettuce
Maple syrup
Milk
Mushrooms
Mustard (spice)
Nutmeg
Orange juice (fresh)
Orange juice (frozen)
Passion fruit
Peaches
Peas boiled
Pepper, white

Peppermint tea
Peppers red
Vegetable
Pickles (dill)
Pineapple juice
Pumpkin canned
Radishes white
Vegetable
Rice white
Saccharine
Scotch whisky
Soy lecithin
Soybean oil
Spearmint tea
Beverage
Spirulina
Supplement
Splenda
Sweetener
Sucralose
Sugar
Tarragon
Turbinado sugar
Turnip
Vanilla
Vanillin
Herb, spice, flavoring
Water chestnuts
Watermelon
Yogurt (commercial)
Zucchini

4. If the vulva feels irritated, pure neem oil, which is vegetable oil derived from the fruit of a tree found in India, may help. You also want to avoid using lubricants, olive oil, or vitamin E because they may promote infections.

5. Intercourse may trigger pain, so alternative ways of having sex must be explored. We recommend that you see a sex therapist to help you with this.

6. We also recommend that you see a trained pelvic physical therapist or women's clinical specialist (www.apta.org/apta/findapt/index.aspx?navID=10737422525) to manually stretch and relax your pelvic muscles. Another good resource is www.pelvicpain.org. You will also need to do your homework. At home, use vaginal dilators (i.e., progressively larger dildos) twice daily to stretch and relieve the tension around your vagina and vulva. You can find hundreds of online stores that sell dildos by doing a Internet search. Two good website sources are vaginismus.com and pelvichealthstore.com.

7. Tricyclic antidepressant medication has been found to decrease pain in patients with vulvodynia. These include amitriptyline, nortriptyline, and similar medications.

8. Injections of one or a combination of medications using local anesthetic with corticosteroids or alcohol, also may help. Injections are more effective than topical forms of these medications.

In some women, light pressure on the vulva from a cotton swab may feel like sharp stabbing or hot scolding pain. Additionally, there may be redness and inflammation in the area of the vaginal opening. This focused area of pain and redness is known as vulvar vestibulitis. If all the previous treatments have been exhausted, then a surgery called a vestibulectomy may provide relief of vulvar pain in six to eight out of ten patients with vulvar vestibulitis. This surgery involves removing the skin and part of the underlying tissue of the vulva and vagina in the areas that are inflamed and painful.

Ovarian cancer

Ovarian cancer is not a diagnosis that one thinks of when thinking about pelvic pain. However, it is something that should be ruled out by your doctor early on in the work up of CPP. Ovarian cancer is known as a silent killer as it is often not caught early (usually diagnosed in stage 3 out of 4 or when it has spread beyond the ovary to other organs in the abdomen). Unlike the Pap smear for cervical cancer, there is no screening test for ovarian cancer. Thus, by the time patients develop symptoms, such as diffuse abdominal pain, increased abdominal girth, and urinary frequency, the cancer has spread beyond the ovary. Use of birth control, the tying of one's tubes, and pregnancy at an early age have all been associated with lowering your risk of ovarian cancer. The symptoms of ovarian cancer can include pelvic/abdominal/back pain, bloating, weight loss, tiredness, constipation, trouble breathing, feeling full soon after eating, and vaginal bleeding.

Since there is no screening test for ovarian cancer, it is important that you see your gynecologist every year for a pelvic exam. If something doesn't feel right during the pelvic exam, then your physician will order a vaginal ultrasound and blood test(s). Usually, the treatment for ovarian cancer involves surgery by a gynecologic oncologist followed by chemotherapy.

Urethral diverticulum

A urethral diverticulum can cause pelvic pain, urinary tract infection, frequency and/or painful urination, dribbling of urine after urination, and pain with intercourse. Occasionally, the diverticulum can become filled with a stone or can become cancerous.

If the urethral diverticulum is causing symptoms, then it must be surgically repaired by a specialist in urogynecology and pelvic reconstructive surgery or a urologist who has experience with this surgical procedure.

Bladder cancer

A person with bladder cancer can have symptoms of pelvic pain, weight loss, lethargy, painful urination, a need to go to the bathroom often, and blood in the urine. The most common risk factors for bladder cancer are smoking, long-term chronic bladder infection or irritation, and chemical exposure at work. Treatment may consist of surgery to remove the tumor (if the cancer is early) along with instillation of chemotherapy into the bladder. However, if the cancer is invasive, treatment could involve removal of the entire bladder, chemotherapy, and radiation. Bladder cancer should be treated by a urologist who has experience in oncology, or a urologic oncologist. (Again, refer to Chapter One, for more specific information regarding finding the best doctor for your specific condition.)

Irritable bowel syndrome

Irritable bowel syndrome (IBS) is a disorder that involves abdominal and pelvic cramping and pain, which is associated with changes in bowel movement (either diarrhea or constipation or both). We do not know what causes IBS, but scientists believe there is an increased sensitivity in the nerves of the bowel (i.e., hypersensitive), which causes an abnormal response of the bowel to normal stimuli. Patients with IBS often have symptoms that may include abdominal discomfort, bloating and gas, straining to defecate, frequency, sensation of incomplete defecation, or passage of mucus. Some people have IBS for periods of time (weeks or months) and then they improve, but the symptoms return. Others have IBS symptoms all the time. IBS has a strong relationship to stress (i.e., IBS gets worse when you have stress in your life). Although they sound similar, IBS is not the same as inflammatory bowel disease, or IBD (also known as ulcerative colitis or Crohn's disease), which is more serious. IBS does not cause harm to your intestines, and it does not lead to colon cancer. Physicians refer to IBS as a diagnosis of exclusion, which means that once all other identifiable conditions (such as Crohn's disease, celiac, infections, cancer, lactose intolerance, etc.) of the bowel have been ruled out by your doctor, then you are diagnosed with IBS. In fact, this diagnosis is the most common reason why patients are sent to a gastroenterologist.

The reason we mention IBS in this chapter, as well as in Chapter Seven when we discuss other gastrointestinal and bowel conditions, is because there is a strong association between CPP and IBS because many women with IBS also have a worsening of their bowel symptoms around the time of ovulation or menstruation.

Emma is a 28-year-old banker who has seen one of us for severe, intermittent lower abdominal and pelvic pain. She says it is an aching type of pain that is all over her abdomen and gets worse around the time of her periods and during ovulation. Her menstrual cycles are regular. Her bowel movements are irregular and alternate between diarrhea and constipation.

Her pain improves after bowel movements. She has tried birth control pills and over-the-counter pain medications, but nothing seems to help.

To establish the diagnosis of IBS, two of the following symptoms must be true for at least 12 weeks out of the year:

1. Abdominal, pelvic pain or discomfort that is relieved with defecation
2. A change in the frequency of your bowel movements
3. A change in your stool's appearance (it becomes hard and lumpy or loose and watery
4. Abdominal or pelvic pain occurs with diarrhea and/or constipation

Patients with IBS fall into three categories. They either have diarrhea or constipation most of the time, or they may alternate between the two. Those who have diarrhea predominant-IBS literally have diarrhea all the time. These individuals usually complain of loose, watery stools one or more times every day, and these bowel movements are difficult to suppress once there is an urge to defecate. This is known as fecal urgency. There are other patients that have constipation predominanr-IBS, meaning they are chronically constipated. These individuals complain of infrequent bowel movements (sometimes only one bowel movement per week), the need to strain, incomplete sensation of evacuation after bowel movements, and cramping during and after bowel movements.

The other category of IBS is made up of those who have diarrhea sometimes and at other times have constipation. These individuals alternate between constipation and diarrhea, sometimes within a single day.

Your doctor may rule out other conditions before he or she can make the diagnosis of IBS. Commonly, colon cancer will be ruled out by performing a blood test to check for anemia and colonoscopy with possible biopsy to look for colon cancer. If you have chronic diarrhea, infection will be ruled out by collecting your stool for culture and for analysis for parasites. To rule-out lactase deficiency (an essential enzyme that digests milk products), your doctor may ask you to eat a lactose-free diet for a period of time to see if your symptoms improve.

Treatment Options for IBS

Once your doctor has determined that you have IBS, then the treatment consists of trying to improve your symptoms through lifestyle changes, including reducing your daily mental, emotional, and physical stress, improving your sleep hygiene (getting enough sleep and sleeping more regularly), and adapting to the Down There diet (see Table 2 and Table 3 for a list of IBS-friendly foods). Meditation, breathing exercises, prayer, yoga, Pilates or tai chi, and getting involved in activities or hobbies are also proven ways to reduce your stress level. (For more information on stress reduction, see Chapter Thirteen.)

IBS is directly related to stress, so it's important to try different ways to relax and reduce stress. Do whichever works best for you and the one that is the most enjoyable! Change your diet to eat more natural fiber, and reduce/eliminate certain foods from your diet (alcohol, caffeine, milk products, chocolate, wheat, certain types of vegetables, spicy foods) (see Table 3). Both of us enjoy spicy foods, so this is difficult advice to give; but if you have IBS, it is wise to reduce your intake of spicy Indian, Thai, Vietnamese, Cajun, and Mexican foods. Finally, medications also may be necessary if the above is not effective. For example, symptoms of bloating and gas may be treated with an over-the-counter gas relief medication such as Beano or Gas-X™ (simethicone). Walking 15 to 30 minutes per day can also make a big difference. Symptoms of diarrhea may be treated with an antidiarrhea agent such as loperamide (be careful not to overdo it as you can easily become constipated). You may also naturally thicken your stools by eating bananas, applesauce, and tapioca. Symptoms of bowel spasm and pain may be treated with medications such as hyoscyamine, dicyclomine, and propantheline. Aerobic exercise may also help.

Table 2. **Down There High-Fiber Diet**

- Choose more fresh fruits and vegetables:

apples	pears
bananas	potatoes
blueberries	prunes
broccoli	raisins
Brussels sprouts	spinach
cantaloupe	strawberries
carrots	sweet potatoes
figs	tomatoes
oranges	zucchini
peaches	

- Choose more whole-grain breads, pastas, and cereals:

All-Bran	oat bran
barley	oatmeal
Bran Flakes	pumpernickel bread
brown rice	raisin bran
granola	whole-grain breads

- Choose more dried beans, peas, nuts, and seeds (as tolerated):

baked beans	split peas
lentils	sunflower seeds
peanuts	walnuts
soy products, such as tofu and textured vegetable protein	

- Choose more snacks that are high in fiber:

  cereal mix with nuts and seeds
  fresh fruit
  fresh vegetables
  popcorn
  whole-grain cereal
  yogurt with bran cereal

- Plan more vegetarian meals:

  bean and rice burritos
  beans and rice
  hummus and pita bread
  pasta with vegetables
  split pea or lentil soup
  vegetable stir fry

Table 3. **The Down There Diet for IBS**

- foods to avoid or foods that cause diarrhea:

bacon	mayonnaise
baked beans	MSG
beer	NutraSweet
broccoli	nuts
cauliflower	processed meats
chocolate	prune juice
coffee, in large quantity	raw fruits
corn	red wine
dried beans	shellfish
fatty foods	sorbitol/mannitol
fructose	soups
garlic	spinach
highly spiced foods	sugar
hot beverages	whole grains
large meals	
licorice	

- Other things that may help relieve diarrhea are as follows:

avocados	pears
boiled white rice	smooth peanut butter
crackers	tapioca
cream of rice	tea (weakly brewed)
Metamucil™	toast
nectars	yogurt with live cultures

Modified from University of Pittsburgh Medical Center (http://www.upmc.com/HealthAtoZ/patienteducation/Documents/IrritableBowelDiet.pdf) and International Pelvic Pain Society: www.pelvicpain.org.

Muscle Pain

The current term for muscle pain related to CPP is myofascial pelvic pain syndrome. Many terms have been used to describe a similar phenomenon, including pelvic floor tension myalgia, coccygodynia, proctalgia fugax, levator ani spasm syndrome, etc. A large number of patients with pelvic pain have spasm and tenderness in their pelvic muscles (see Chapter One for section on female anatomy). We do not know why this occurs, but anxiety and stress are likely to contribute to tensing your pelvic muscles as they are to causing tense neck, shoulder, and scalp muscles.

Need a massage? Essentially, myofascial pelvic pain is a chronic charley horse in your pelvic muscles. When a muscle goes into spasm, it not only becomes contracted and tender but it also becomes less useful to your body because it is weaker and doesn't relax; and thus, it doesn't function normally. In turn, the muscles adjacent to the muscle spasm have to work harder to compensate for their neighbors inadequate performance, and this causes the neighboring muscles to also become shorter, firmer, and painful as well. Pain signals from these muscles travel to the spinal cord and then to the brain to alert the person that there is pain in the pelvic area. Often, the sensory nerves that carry the pain signal into the spinal cord synapse in the same area of the spinal cord that also receives signals from your pelvic organs such as the bladder, rectum, vagina, and uterus. There may be crisscrossing of these signals and your brain may interpret the pain as emerging from one of your pelvic organs.

For this reason, women with pelvic muscle pain may have symptoms such as rectal pain, constipation, pain with defecation, frequency of urination, bladder pain and interstitial cystitis symptoms, vaginal and vulvar discomfort, and pain with intercourse. These patients may also have pain in other areas such lower abdominal wall, buttocks, and thigh pain. In fact, treatment of lower abdominal wall tender muscles (trigger points) can improve pelvic pain. Each tender spot is located within a tight band of muscle. Sometimes an old surgical scar can be the source of myofascial problems. Pain and tenderness is not the only symptom as some patients only complain of cramping, burning, aching, or heaviness in their pelvic area.

Nerve pain

The most common type of nerve pain leading to CPP is called pudendal neuralgia. Injury to the pudendal nerve may result from a history of trauma such as vaginal delivery, previous surgery, heavy lifting, or from a fall. This type of pain is often burning, numbing, or tingling; the pain is worsened by sitting in a chair but may improve with sitting on the toilet seat or a donut cushion. The diagnosis is made when injection of the pudendal nerve with medications relieves the pain, even for a short duration.

The most appropriate initial treatment for myofascial pelvic pain is pelvic floor physical therapy. A physical therapist with an advanced degree and experience in pelvic muscle treatment or women's clinical specialist utilizes different techniques to mobilize, stretch, relax, and strengthen the muscles in and around the pelvis. This treatment usually takes less than an hour and should be done weekly for at least eight weeks. In addition to providing therapy for muscles on the outside of the pelvis, the physical therapist will need to manipulate the muscles inside your pelvis while you are lying on your back with your thighs open. In fact, the internal muscle mobilization is key to successful treatment of myofascial pelvic pain.

There are anecdotal reports that diazepam (Valium) or lorazepam (Ativan) and baclofen (Lioresal) suppositories, placed in the vagina, may take the edge off of the pelvic floor pain and spasm, especially at night. Although the compounded gels of these medications are easier to take than placing a tablet inside the vagina, the latter can be cheaper.

In addition, two oral medications have been shown to be effective for treatment of chronic pain throughout the body, including gabapentin (Neurontin). This medication can be started at 300 mg once at bedtime and over a short period of time should be increased to three times daily. Often, patients with CPP may need higher doses of this medication to achieve optimal pain relief. The medication can be increased to up to 2,400 mg daily as long as you are able to tolerate the side effects. These include stomach upset, dizziness, sleepiness, and blurry vision. Another medication that is effective for chronic pain is called pregabalin (Lyrica). In some patients, this is more effective than Neurontin. However, there may be other side effects with Lyrica. These include forgetfulness, fogginess, dry mouth, dizziness, stomach upset, and weight gain.

Trigger point injections are useful for those who cannot tolerate physical therapy or as an adjunct to physical therapy. Usually, a local anesthetic agent by itself is used at first. Sometimes a cocktail of medication that includes a local anesthetic, botulinum toxin (Botox), and a corticosteroid is mixed together and injected into the tender points. Trigger point injections are effective and may be even more effective when they are followed by physical therapy. Injections allow deeper manipulation of the pelvic muscles by the physical therapist. For those who failed pelvic floor physical therapy, lack sufficient progress, or for whom the trigger point injections do not last, consideration can be given to adding Botox to the mixture.

Sacral nerve stimulation (neuromodulation) may provide temporary relief of pain in patients with CPP, especially if the CPP is associated with voiding problems. This treatment is described in more detail in Chapter Four.

A final option for pain associated with pudendal neuralgia is surgery where an incision is made over the buttocks area, muscles are separated, and the pudendal nerve is decompressed and scar tissue around the nerve is removed.

Psychiatric

Studies show that 40 to 50 percent of women with CPP have a history of sexual or physical abuse and are at risk for developing somatization disorder, a psychiatric condition in which a person has multiple physical complaints that are experienced as real, but no physical cause can be found. Because pain is a matter of perception, it can be dramatically modified in patients who have been subjected to sexual or physical abuse. The pain can also be experienced differently in someone who is depressed.

One patient, Madeline, a 34-year-old mother of two, described experiencing pelvic pain for the past six years. Her pain interferes with her ability to enjoy activities that she once enjoyed, and it interferes with her marital intimacy. She also has low energy, poor appetite, and does not sleep well. She is unable to concentrate on her work. She has lost 15 pounds even though she is not on a diet. She often cries and snaps at family members. She has been feeling this way for several months. She has had a complete workup, which includes blood tests, CT scans, MRI, physical therapy consultation—and nothing seems to explain her pelvic pain. Based on her symptoms, she fits the definition of major depression. In Madeline's case, the pelvic pain and depression are interrelated.

Some antidepressant medications known as tricylclic antidepressants (e.g., amitriptyline, desipramine, and doxepin) as well as serotonin-norepinephrine reuptake inhibitors have been found to be useful in treatment of certain pain conditions, especially vulvodynia and CPP that is associated with underlying depression. The natural course of depression is six to 12 months, and treatment should be continued for at least that long. We recommend combination of medicine along with psychotherapy with a psychologist or therapist who has experience treating pain disorders.

Form a Multidisciplinary Team to Get the Help You Need

Treating CPP is one of the most challenging aspects of being a doctor—not only because it is difficult to diagnose properly but also challenging to treat. It is no surprise that patients with CPP sometimes are subconsciously sent away from doctors' practices. Alternatively, many with CPP become dissatisfied with lack of a diagnosis or with the inadequacy of treatment and thus they become doctor shop-a-holics. Most women with CPP have seen more than five doctors before an accurate diagnosis has been made and appropriate therapy initiated.

If you have CPP and do any of these very understandable behaviors, don't worry! We understand you. Many in your situation do the same. It's not easy living with the constant pain and agony that you have dealt with for so long. Your condition is legitimate. It's not just in your head. You need to find the right doctor, one who understands what we've been discussing so far. How do you do that? The doctor who treats your pelvic pain doesn't have to be a genius or world famous. The right doctor must have the willingness, knowledge, and compassion to go through all that will be necessary to manage your pain. Your doctor should be a good listener. If the doctor interrupts you after a few seconds of the first encounter, you likely do not have the right doctor, and you should politely terminate the visit and seek out another opinion.

Your doctor should be ready to coordinate your care with other healthcare professionals, as no doctor can be a Superman when it comes to treating CPP. The right doctor will properly counsel you so that you don't have unreasonable expectations and think that a cure or a miracle is going to happen, because neither one exists for CPP. Try to find a doctor who is part of a multidisciplinary team of doctors with other healthcare professionals who work together to address your pain (see Table 4). Your team will need to individualize therapy for you. This will increase your chances of success. We hope this chapter has helped you. Good luck on your journey to finding relief from pain.

Table 4. **Multidisciplinary Approach**

Patient	Self-help, friends, family, others who have your specific condition (after you have a diagnosis)
Physician	Obstetrician/gynecologist, urologist, urogynecologist, female pelvic medicine and reconstructive surgeon, physical medicine and rehabilitation specialist, psychiatrist, pain medicine specialist, neurologist, gastroenterologist, rheumatologist, sexual medicine specialist, sports medicine practitioner
Therapists and practitioners	Women's clinical specialist, sexual therapist, couples therapist, psychologist, pharmacist, nurse practitioner, physician assistant

The Bottom Line

CPP is a common and disabling condition that affects more than 45 million Americans. You don't have to continue to suffer in silence. Help is available. Find a doctor who is understanding and is knowledgeable, and he/she will provide you with treatment and relief.

Chapter Six

When Something Down There Is Wrong with Your Cycle: Premenstrual Syndrome

Is there a time in the month when you feel like you are just off? Does your body feel achy and bloated? Do you feel irritable and tired?

Let's start by asking some questions: At a certain time in the month, do you do any of the following:

- Cry for no apparent reason or at silly commercials?
- Crave sweets?
- Feel swollen?
- Remain silent so you don't offend people?
- Become angry for no apparent reason?
- Act impatiently?
- Offend people in your household?
- Feel more sensitive than usual?
- Stress out your boyfriend or husband?
- Get grumpy and cranky?

In response to these cyclical changes in behavior, does your partner suddenly agree with everything you say? Do the people in your house know when your period is coming? Do you mix chocolate into your omelettes? Do people drive you crazy?

If even a few of these descriptions ring true for you at a certain time each month, then you may be suffering from a medical condition known as premenstrual syndrome, or PMS.

PMS is real. It's not imaginary; it's not an exaggeration. And it occurs irrespective of socioeconomic status or culture. In the past, some doctors believed that the term *PMS* was just medicalization of a natural phenomenon. However, we no longer believe this to be true. PMS is a genuine medical condition that comprises the mood and physical symptoms that many women begin to experience from days to two weeks before their menstrual period. These symptoms may last up to two weeks and may even continue through the beginning of the menstrual period.

To be considered *PMS*, the timing of these symptoms is important. For example in the typical 28-day cycle, if symptoms occur during days 5 to 12 of the cycle, then by definition, it is not considered PMS. The symptoms have to occur after ovulation and during the luteal phase (second half of the cycle) to be considered PMS (see PMS definition box on the next page). The symptoms of PMS fall along a wide spectrum. Most women, who think they are PMSing, describe mild symptoms that consist of only one or a few nuisances, such as bloating and tenderness and swelling of the breasts, constipation, and weight gain. Usually these nuisance symptoms do not interfere with women's lives, but for some, even one of the symptoms can be so severe and disrupting, that this time of the month overshadows their lives. Take for instance Tracy, a forty-five-year-old mother of three boys. Every month and starting about two weeks before her last period, she begins to "get the downs." "I just don't feel like myself. I want to hide in my room, I don't want to work out. All I want to do is sleep, but I can't. My legs hurt, my ankles swell. I'm a mess." But for years, Tracy did not know that these symptoms were part of PMS. Now, she is a candidate for fluoxetine.

Tracy is not alone. For many women, PMS symptoms can be so severe, their whole lives are oriented around waiting for it to happen, enduring the discomfort when it's present, and recovering from it after it has passed. Their PMS takes away their energy, focus, and sense of control over their lives.

In another case, Jocelyn is a 35-year-old woman who, for the last four years, has experienced persistent anger, irritability, and inability to concentrate about one week before her periods begin. All these symptoms go away as soon as her menses start. Her PMS has been interfering with her ability to do her job because she is not able to interact normally with her coworkers or pay attention to her work. "They just irritate me," she says.

Her mom says she cries for no apparent reason and is very sensitive a few days out of the month. Her husband thinks the world of her, but admits that the only fights they have ever had during their 10-year marriage have always occurred during "that time of the month." Now, to avoid conflict, her husband has learned to work late during those trying times.

Do You Have PMS?

There is no single test to diagnose PMS. To be considered PMS, the symptoms must have the following characteristics, and they must interfere with your normal activities or cause problems with your social, parental, marital, school, work, or personal relationships. If the following characteristics describe what you go through every month, then you have PMS:

- Behavioral or mood symptoms may include anxiety, moodiness, irritability, confusion, social withdrawal, trouble getting to sleep, sleeping too much, difficulty concentrating, appetite changes, food cravings, changes in sexual desire, forgetfulness and depression.
- Physical symptoms may consist of bloating, fatigue, breast tenderness, headache, dizziness, swelling, joint and muscle pain, heart palpitations, abdominal pain, and weight gain.
- You experience both these types of symptoms each and every month, for at least two consecutive menstrual cycles.
- Your symptoms generally occur several days to more than a week before your period starts and may continue for a few days after you start your period.

When PMS Spirals Out of Control

We distinguish this type of PMS from a more severe, incapacitating form of PMS called premenstrual dysphoric disorder, or PMDD. This is a psychiatric diagnosis that is a form of depression, which occurs strictly for a period of time each month and then disappears until the next menstrual cycle.

Joanna is a 30-year-old woman who believes that every month she goes through severe depression for about a week, which then lifts within the first two days of her periods. She says it is awful and "some months I think about killing myself." She says during that one week of hell, she is not able to concentrate, she can't get a full night's sleep because she wakes up early in the morning, she loses her appetite, has low energy level, and has difficulty performing her normal daily activities. She has been fired from three jobs because she is not able to perform well during that time of the month. She has trouble taking care of her four-year-old son during those times. She isolates herself from the world and doesn't even like to be around her husband. But then, like flash, within a couple of days of the start of her period, she feels normal again.

In order for you to have PMDD, you must have five or more of the above symptoms (especially the behavioral symptoms), and these have to occur most of the time during only the second half of the menstrual cycle. In other words, patients diagnosed with PMDD fit the definition of depression, but these symptoms occur only during a period of time in the second half of the menstrual cycle.

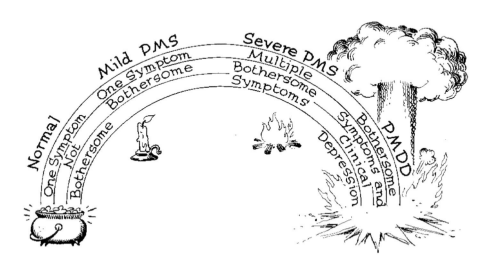

A Closer Look at PMS

Although PMS symptoms can start with your very first menstrual cycle, they may become more severe or bothersome as you get older. In fact, most women who see their doctors for treatment of PMS do so after age 30.

Many women mistakenly assume that stress can cause PMS. Let us put your fears at rest: if you have a high-stress job and your life involves juggling many balls, you are not more likely to experience PMS symptoms. However, having severe PMS symptoms does make coping with stress more difficult.

The causes of PMS are not well understood, but we do know that female hormones (estrogen and progesterone) do not cause PMS. If hormones were the cause of PMS, then all women would have PMS. Doctors and scientists believe that in certain vulnerable women, the fluctuation of these normal female hormones affects sensitive body and brain tissues. The brain of a person experiencing PMS is sensitive to the fluctuating hormones, and this leads to changes in the chemical messengers or neurotransmitters, especially serotonin, which affects mood.

The frustrating part of PMS, for both patient and doctor, is that we don't know what makes a person more vulnerable or sensitive to these normal hormonal fluctuations that occur throughout the month and over the lifespan.

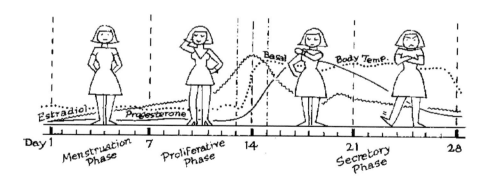

What to Do When You Have PMS

By keeping a symptom diary on your monthly calendar, you can determine whether you fit the definition of PMS described above.

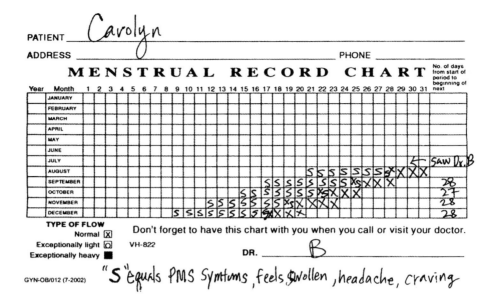

PATIENT _Carolyn_

ADDRESS _____ PHONE _____

MENSTRUAL RECORD CHART

No. of days from start of period to beginning of next

Year	Month	1	2	3	4	5	6	7	8	9	10	11	12	13	14	15	16	17	18	19	20	21	22	23	24	25	26	27	28	29	30	31	
	JANUARY																																
	FEBRUARY																																
	MARCH																																
	APRIL																																
	MAY																																
	JUNE																																
	JULY																																⌐ SAW Dr. B
	AUGUST																		S	S	S	S	S	S	S	S	X	X	X	X			
	SEPTEMBER																S	S	S	S	S	S	S	S	S	X	X	X			28		
	OCTOBER														S	S	S	S	S	S	X	X	X	X					27			
	NOVEMBER												S	S	S	S	S	S	X	X	X	X							28			
	DECEMBER								S	S	S	S	S	S	S	X	X	X											28				

TYPE OF FLOW

Don't forget to have this chart with you when you call or visit your doctor.

Normal ☒
Exceptionally light ⊡   VH-822
Exceptionally heavy ■

DR. _____ B _____

GYN-OB/012 (7-2002)

"S" equals PMS Symptoms, feels swollen, headache, craving

Some women, who are not significantly impacted by their symptoms, don't bother going to see a doctor. In fact, if you have only mild symptoms that don't interfere with your life, there is no need to consult your physician, and you just need to recognize this as a normal part of the menstrual cycle.

However, if you have multiple symptoms, the symptoms are interfering with your quality of life, or you believe you have PMDD, then your doctor—your gynecologist or family doctor—may be able to help you. If your symptoms are severe enough to interfere with your lifestyle or your relationships, one of the first things that your doctor will do is to rule out other medical or psychiatric condition(s) that can be masquerading as PMS.

More importantly, your doctor will try to differentiate your symptoms from major depression. Your doctor may rule out other underlying medical or psychiatric conditions that can be worsened during that time of the month. Your doctor will also do a physical exam and may order a few blood tests (such as thyroid stimulating hormone level for thyroid disease, complete blood count for anemia, and basic metabolic panel for electrolytes and kidney function). Perhaps the most important action that your doctor will take is to give you information about PMS, which in itself can relieve your anxiety.

We often see patients who have been going through significant symptoms of PMS and were told by friends and family that they have PMS and not to worry. But they often have thought to themselves that "maybe there is something wrong with me. Do I have a psychiatric problem? Do I have a personality disorder?" After seeing one of us and plotting a monthly diary of symptoms (as shown on the previous page) in relationship to their periods and being diagnosed with PMS, finally they felt a sense of relief to know why they feel so out of whack during part of each and every month.

Indeed, having your doctor explain the condition and reassure you that this is common makes many women feel better.

Other Medical Conditions Affected by PMS

Conditions such as anxiety, panic disorder, migraines, seizures, and irritable bowel syndrome may be magnified by PMS, and the treatment for PMS may reduce the symptoms of these conditions as well.

Do-It-Yourself Treatments for PMS

If you have PMS and are nodding your head as you read this chapter and wish that you didn't have to deal with the symptoms every month, there is hope. There are some simple treatments that you can employ at home to alleviate your PMS symptoms:

- Diet—maintain your blood sugar throughout the day. By eating breakfast, regular meals, and healthy snacks, such as fresh fruit and fresh vegetables, throughout the day, you will keep a steady blood sugar level. This will avoid a drop in your blood sugar level, which can worsen your PMS symptoms.
- Some scientific evidence suggests that specially formulated carbohydrate drinks, such as PMS Escape, may help with mood and food craving symptoms of PMS. The blend of simple and complex carbohydrates promotes an increase in the blood ratio of the amino acid, tryptophan, which is a precursor to serotonin, thus

making it easier for the brain to make serotonin. Our advice when it comes to carbohydrates is to avoid overloading on simple sugars that are found in cake, cookies, candy, and ice cream. Instead, eat complex carbohydrates such as whole grains, brown rice, oatmeal, fruits, vegetables, barley, and beans.

- Exercise—Although exercise in itself has not been proven to treat PMS, it has so many beneficial effects on your health and on the reduction of stress and anxiety that we highly recommend it.
- Relaxation and stress reduction—PMS can be worsened by stress, which means that stress reduction can be helpful in the treatment of PMS and many other medical conditions described in this book. See Chapter Thirteen on stress and how to reduce it so that your symptoms down there are more manageable.
- Chasteberry (also discussed in Chapter Nine)—The fruit of the Chasteberry tree (*Vitex agnus castus*) has been suggested as a natural treatment agent for mild PMS symptoms. Strong scientific evidence that it actually works is currently lacking, but one study did show a positive impact. We recommend taking two 400 mg capsules twice daily, preferably with meals.
- Calcium or magnesium—Either calcium or magnesium by itself, not combined, has been suggested for treatment of mild PMS, but there is a weak scientific evidence to support it. However, since they are inexpensive and in moderate doses (calcium 1,200 mg or magnesium 600 mg per day) are not harmful, we suggest you consider this as a nonmedical treatment for PMS. You can also get calcium in your diet by eating yogurt, cheese, low-fat cow-or fortified soy milk, and fortified juices.
- Vitamin B6 or vitamin E—Pyridoxine, or vitamin B6, has been suggested for treatment of mild PMS. Vitamin E 400 IU/day has also been suggested. Although scientific evidence of their efficacy is weak, we recommend supplemental vitamin B6 or vitamin E as long as high doses are not taken. For example, daily vitamin B6 in excess of 100 mg may be harmful to your nerves, and therefore, we recommend taking only 50 to 100 mg per day.
- St. John's Wort—There is new evidence that daily St. John's Wort may improve some of the symptoms of PMS (also discussed in Chapter Nine).
- Over-the-counter medications—Medications such as Midol, Pamprin, Premsyn have been marketed for menstrual cramps and

PMS symptoms. Depending on the formulation, they may contain a pain reliever such as acetaminophen or naprosyn for cramps, an antihistamine such as diphenhydramine or pyrilamine to help you sleep, and diuretic or water pill, which may help with the sensation of bloating. Women should be cautioned about using combination products, which may provide inadequate doses of some ingredients and excessive doses of others. If nonprescription preparations are used, single-ingredient products (i.e., vitamins or analgesics) are preferred.

Asking Your Doctor for Help

If these holistic approaches to alleviating your PMS do not work, there are some medications that can treat your PMS.

- SSRIs—This class of antidepressant medications, which are defined as selective serotonin reuptake inhibitors (SSRIs), have been used to treat multiple medical conditions, but have been specifically shown to be effective for severe PMS and PMDD. An SSRI can be taken in several ways. A woman with PMS can take the medication only during the second half of her menstrual cycle each month and may stop the medication at the onset of her periods. Another method of taking SSRI for PMS is to take it on a daily basis throughout the entire cycle. This second method, or daily use, may be more effective. Common side effects of SSRIs include abdominal upset, nausea, jitteriness, headache, trouble sleeping, and inability to have an orgasm or reduced sexual interest. However, a low dose taken in the morning is usually effective for treatment of PMS and has only minimal side effects. The most common SSRIs and their recommended dose for the treatment of severe PMS include the following: fluoxetine 20 mg (Serafem, Prozac), paroxetine 25 mg (Paxil), sertraline 50 mg (Zoloft), and citalopram 20 mg (Celexa). Another type of antidepressant medication that has been shown to treat PMS is venlafaxine (Effexor). This medication not only modulates serotonin levels in the brain, but it also changes another chemical messenger known as norepinephrine. If the conservative treatments of supplements and vitamins described above fail, then SSRIs are the best option. If you have tried one of these SSRIs and it has not helped, then you should ask your doctor to switch you to a different SSRI. And if you have tried multiple SSRIs without relief, then your doctor may put you on a low-dose antianxiety medication such as alprazolam. This drug will calm you but it may also make you sleepy and has potential to be habit-forming.

- Birth control pills—Some women with PMS or PMDD have relief from their PMS symptoms by taking birth control pills. Yaz, the low-dose pill, has been approved in the United States for the treatment of PMDD. This birth control pill contains a low dose of estrogen (ethinyl estradiol, 20 micrograms) plus a special type of progestin, (Drosperinone, 3 mg), which may be responsible for its success. Usually, women take pills containing hormones for 21 days in their cycle and take an inactive, sugar pill the remaining seven days of their cycle. With Yaz, however, the hormone-free (sugar pill) days have been shortened to four days.

- Spironolactone (Aldactone)—Spironolactone is a water pill or diuretic that has been prescribed for various medical conditions such as swelling in the legs and treatment of high blood pressure. There is good scientific evidence showing that 100 mg of spironolactone, taken every day during the two weeks before your period may reduce both physical and behavioral symptoms of PMS.

- Gonadotropin releasing hormone agonists (GnRH agonists)—By artificially inducing menopause with drugs such as leuprolide (Lupron), we can eliminate estrogen and progesterone by shutting down the ovaries, production of these two hormones for a period of time. Temporary menopause may improve many of the physical symptoms of PMS. However, this does come at a price. The side effects of leuprolide include severe hot flashes and bone loss if used for a long period of time such as several years. Because of its effect on the bone, leuprolide should not be taken for a long period of time. When leuprolide is taken for more than six months, your doctor will add back hormones either estrogen or progesterone in order to protect your bones from the osteoporotic effects of leuprolide.

- Danazol—This drug is a type of hormone that has male-hormone-like effects on the body. In sufficient doses it also prevents the ovaries from producing estrogen and progesterone and relieves PMS symptoms. Danazol does, however, have side effects such as unwanted hair growth, acne, oily skin, and weight gain, and it can cause damage to the liver. It may also cause hot flashes, but usually these side effects are much less severe than those caused by leuprolide.

- Surgery for PMS—Surgery has been done in the past for severe PMS but it should only be considered as the last resort. If you are finished having children, then you should talk to your doctor about this option.

PMS Treatment Myths

Keep in mind that there are some ineffective treatments for PMS. These include *Gingko bilboa*, evening primrose oil, and gamma linolenic acid (GLA). Despite the claims, these supplements are not helpful for PMS symptoms. Some other classes of antidepressant medications such as monamine oxidase inhibitors such as Selegeline or moclobemide; tricyclic antidepressants, such as imipramine and nortriptyline; lithium; and progesterone by itself are not effective for the treatment of PMS.

The Bottom Line

If you have PMS and the symptoms are creating havoc in your life, then you should consider speaking with your gynecologist or primary care doctor about receiving some form of treatment. We would recommend starting with dietary changes and exercise. These actions are usually effective for many women. However, if these supportive therapies do not control your symptoms then you should consider seeing your doctor and requesting a prescription for an SSRI. If you've tried at least two different SSRIs and none have helped, then you may need more potent medications. You may either need to take an anti-anxiety medication or shut off your ovaries with a GnRH agonist such as leuprolide. Your doctor will help you figure out the best course of action.

The bottom line is that you don't have to allow PMS to wreak havoc on your life. Help is available for all who suffer from PMS.

Chapter Seven

When It Gets Really Embarrassing Down There: Bowel Control Disorder

"I am absolutely humiliated."

"I've never been more embarrassed in my life."

"I don't think I can even leave the house again."

These are just a few of the many comments we have heard over the years in response to problems experienced in the bowels. Indeed, there is no condition that we see in our offices that is a source of more anxiety, embarrassment, and depression than fecal incontinence or accidental loss of stool or feces. Fecal incontinence is perhaps the leading cause of a woman's loss of confidence and self-esteem and affects women of all ages. These are women who become so fearful of having an accident in public that they begin to withdraw socially, emotionally, and sexually. They become frozen in fear, no longer able to relax and lead their normal lives. Bowel control disorder (BCD), or fecal incontinence, is one of the greatest maladies that can occur down there.

The most common cause for BCD is trauma from vaginal childbirth. Another common cause is surgical trauma (such as hemorrhoid surgery), type 2 diabetes, decreased rectal compliance (typically from radiation treatment), impaired rectal sensation (as a result of a spinal cord injury), and constipation that leads to stool impaction. But there's good news and more good news. First, it is not as common as the other conditions we have discussed; and second, and most importantly, it is treatable.

Daily or weekly episodes of fecal incontinence occur in about 2 percent of the adult population and in about 7 percent of healthy independent-living adults over the age of 65. But these rates are an underestimation since this embarrassing condition is often underreported. The incidence of the problem increases with infirmity, and a third of elderly people who are hospitalized or in residential care are incontinent of stool. But for those women who are affected, it can be an embarrassing nuisance that significantly lessens the quality of their lives.

Where the Problem Starts

By becoming a bit more familiar with the anatomy of the rectum, you will get a better picture of how the problem of fecal incontinence can begin.

Food is taken in through the mouth and then digested in the stomach and intestines. Food is broken down into the nutrients that the body needs and is absorbed from the intestines into the bloodstream. The waste travels to the colon where water is absorbed, and the waste remains until it is socially acceptable to expel the waste, or feces, into the toilet. The muscles in the rectum remain contracted to facilitate the storage of the fecal contents until it is time to use the restroom. The rectum consists of a set of muscles, or sphincters, that contract to keep the feces within the body. When the rectum becomes distended with feces, nerves supplying the sphincters send a message to the brain indicating whether the distension is due to gas or to semisolid feces. Pretty smart set of muscles! Another amazing function of the rectum is that the walls of the rectum can distend and stretch, which allows a woman to hold the stool for a longer period of time until she can reach a toilet and empty her rectum of the feces. When the brain senses that the distension is due to feces and the time is appropriate to empty the rectum, the muscles or sphincters will relax, the anus opens, and the fecal contents are expelled.

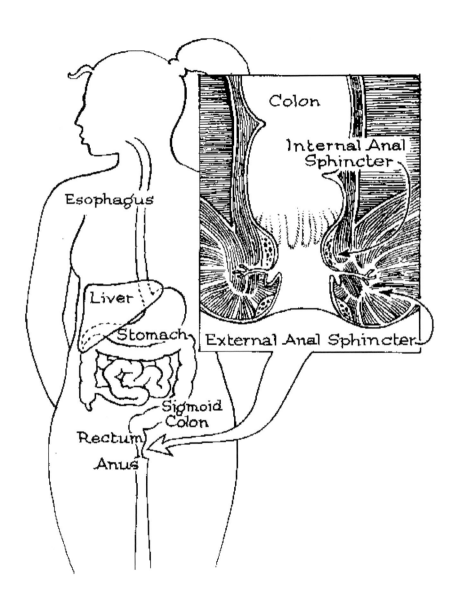

The Smartness of Your Sphincter

A renowned proctologist, WC Bornemeier, describes the "cleverness" of the rectal sphincter as follows: "The average fart is a wondrous event. Let me demonstrate with a little experiment. Interlock the fingers of your two hands tightly together to make a little cup, with your palms facing upwards. Imagine that in the cup of your hands you have some water, some floating solids and some gas. Imagine the whole system is under pressure. Now try to open one of your fingers in such a way that you release only the gas, without letting any solid or liquid squirt out. I really doubt that any device made by the human race could do this task—and keep on doing it for seventy years. This is the magnificent job that your anal sphincter does some ten times per day, and usually without making a mistake. It apparently can tell whether its owner is alone or with someone, whether standing up or sitting down, and whether its owner has his (her) pants on or off. No other muscle in the body is such a protector of the dignity of man (woman), yet so ready to come to his (her) relief." Let the truth be told; this kind of reasoning makes one believe in intelligent design!

A Jewish Prayer

Most individuals learn social control of the anal muscles by the age of two-and-a-half to three and can then throw away their diapers. However, when those muscles fail to close when they are supposed to remain closed, fecal incontinence occurs. It is interesting to note that observant Jews have a prayer that they recite before they go to the restroom, which translates as, "Dear Lord, thank you for opening my valves when they are supposed to open and that they remain closed when they are supposed to remain shut." We think it is fascinating that more than 3,000 years ago these wise, ancient people understood the importance of sphincters and muscles and never took them for granted.

Causes of Fecal Incontinence

When your plumbing down there is working correctly:

- The nerves from the rectum to the brain are intact;
- The rectum is well supported by pelvic floor muscles;
- The rectum can fill adequately;
- You have a sense of rectal fullness; and
- You have the ability to reach the toilet in a timely fashion.

However, if any of the above are injured, nonfunctioning, or damaged, BCD can happen.

As we've seen, pregnancy and especially vaginal childbirth can place a significant stress on the pelvic floor muscles. Childbirth can stretch, weaken, and sometimes tear these pelvic floor muscles, as well as cause damage to nerves that supply the rectum and anal sphincter. Surgical incisions, episiotomy, and use of forceps to expedite vaginal delivery can also cause injury to this area. These injuries that occur during procedures used to facilitate childbirth can cause damage to the muscles; the results of these injuries may show up decades later, and thus childbirth damage is the number one cause of fecal incontinence. Risk factors for injury include multiple childbirths, delivery of large babies, or preexisting conditions affecting the rectum, such as hemorrhoids. These rectal injuries are one of the most common causes of fecal incontinence.

Another common condition that can result in fecal incontinence is pelvic organ prolapse, as we discussed in Chapter Two. Prolapse occurs when an organ such as the bladder, uterus, or rectum moves out of place or slides in on itself. For instance, the rectum can displace and bulge into the vagina, this is called rectocele.

It is a paradox that constipation is a common yet treatable cause of BCD: constipation leads to fecal impaction, which then causes fecal incontinence. This happens when a woman has been constipated for a long time and the unpassed fecal matter has become so large that the rectum and large intestines are overstretched. As a result, these organs lose their tone and ability to propel or squeeze the stool out of the body. Now liquid feces above the obstructing ball passes around the obstruction and exits without permission, resulting in fecal incontinence.

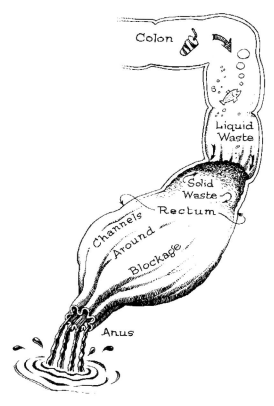

Stool Impaction

Chronic diarrhea can also be a cause of BCD. Usually chronic diarrhea is caused by medical conditions such as irritable bowel syndrome, lactose intolerance, Crohn's disease, and ulcerative colitis. A person with unexplained diarrhea for a long period of time should have a colonoscopy and a blood test (metabolic panel) to rule out serious conditions (such as ulcerative colitis, Crohn's disease, or cancer). More common causes of diarrhea are usually of limited duration. These can be due to viral or bacterial causes such as traveler's diarrhea and usually subside in a few days after the offending organism is purged from the body and you have a ruined vacation as you spend most of the day in bed or on the toilet. Even hemorrhoids, which are common during pregnancy and after menopause, can prevent a good seal to not allow feces to leak out of the rectum.

Drugs, medications, and certain foods and supplements can also cause diarrhea, including caffeine, artificial sweeteners, too much alcohol, and sweets. Supplements such as vitamin C in large doses and niacin can cause diarrhea. We also want to point out that chronic use of laxatives to maintain daily bowel habits can result in fecal incontinence. So beware of that connection!

Any surgical procedure in the pelvic area or colon and anus, such as for a rectovaginal fistula (a connection between the rectum and the vagina), hemorrhoids or rectal abscesses, can also cause muscular damage and weaken the rectal sphincter resulting in BCD. Any surgery in the pelvis or on the large intestines that result in scarring and narrowing of the large intestine and rectum may reduce the capacity to stretch and store feces, which can result in BCD. Women who are treated for rectal cancer often have injuries to the rectal sphincters or to the nerves that supply the sphincters. The muscles are then unable to keep the feces inside the body, causing the woman to lose control. Radiation to the pelvis can also cause injury to the large intestines, the nerves, and the sphincters resulting in BCD.

Damage to the nerves that supply the large intestines and especially to the rectum and the rectal sphincters can also result in fecal incontinence. These nerves can be injured by childbirth, straining when having a bowel movement, spinal cord injury, and stroke. Diseases that affect these nerves, such as diabetes and multiple sclerosis, and cause nerve damage, all can be a factor leading to BCD.

You Can Find Treatment!

Although BCD significantly impacts a woman's quality of life and can be a source of reclusive behavior and social isolation, help is available, and new treatments are on the horizon. These options can greatly improve the symptoms in most women and cure the problem in some afflicted by this condition.

Continence healthcare professionals and specialized nutritionists and dietitians can advise you about dietary changes that might enhance your bowel health or alleviate symptoms. As with most medical conditions affecting both men and women, a healthy lifestyle can help those with fecal incontinence. Also, obesity and excessive weight can place added stress on the pelvic floor muscles, and women who are over their ideal body weight should consider a weight loss program.

Just as behavioral therapy can be of assistance in women with urinary incontinence, behavior modification is a conservative treatment option in women with fecal incontinence. You can train yourself to defecate at certain times of the day. For example, either ritualized bowel habit or stimulated defecation can help alleviate fecal incontinence. Some women use their natural gastrocolic reflex after an adequate breakfast and coffee to stimulate defecation, where food and fluids in the stomach will trigger the colon and rectum to contract. Use of a suppository or enema can also encourage emptying of the contents of your bowel and rectum in the privacy of your home and under controlled conditions before you go out and about. When the colon and rectum are empty, there is a smaller chance of BCD!

You can also train the anal sphincter to hold tight and extend the period between defecations. This is not an instant cure as it takes weeks before results become noticeable. This is not easy to do, but with dedication, it can be done.

Stress reduction can also help women with fecal incontinence. Just as stress can affect many conditions down there, fecal incontinence is one of those conditions that appears to be closely tied to stress. Emotional stress leads to tension in the pelvic floor muscles and in the abdominal muscles. Added tension in the abdomen and pelvis leads to additional pressure and increased bowel activity, thus promoting urgency of defecation and fecal incontinence. Stress reduction techniques consisting of meditation, yoga, exercise, and sleep are all helpful. (For more tips on stress reduction, see Chapter Thirteen.)

Also helpful for those women who have fecal incontinence is to join one of the many support groups. A strong support system with family, friends, and others who suffer from the same condition can be so helpful in regaining your confidence and self-esteem. With a support group, you will learn that you are not alone and that others who have the same problem will share their coping mechanisms. Resources for these support groups include (http://www.experienceproject.com, http://www.aboutincontinence.org/, and https://www.inspire.com/conditions/fecal-incontinence/.

Stop smoking. Nicotine, the active ingredient in cigarettes can increase the motility of the intestines, which can shorten the time from food entering the intestines until it is processed and exits the body. This is referred to as transit time. Many women are looking for motivations to stop smoking, and if nicotine's impact on the intestines and colon is contributing to fecal incontinence, then it is important that you stop smoking as soon as possible.

As you know, pelvic floor exercises or Kegel exercises are effective for treating stress urinary incontinence, and are also effective for improving the tone of the anal sphincter. (See Chapter Two for instructions on performing Turbo Kegel exercises.) We recommend that women do 7 reps, 7 times per day, and seven days a week. You can do the exercises almost at any time, they do not require any equipment, and results occur in just a few weeks. If you don't get good results on your own, then a trained physical therapist or women's clinical specialist can be very helpful. To find one near you, go to www.apta.org.

Biofeedback is an effective treatment for BCD. It can be used in conjunction with Kegel exercises. A device is inserted into the rectum, which is attached to a computer and can measure the voluntary muscle contraction of the anal sphincter or rectum. With this in place, women can see and even hear their muscles contract on a computer screen, which shows a graph of the contraction and the sound of the muscles contracting using sound amplification. Biofeedback can also aid in improving sensation so that your rectum is able to sense smaller and smaller stool loads inside it. This can lead to greater awareness of your bowel contents and thus give enough time to contract your pelvic muscles in order to prevent an accident. Another nonsurgical treatment is dietary modification. Continence healthcare professionals, nutritionists, and dietitians can advise you about dietary changes that might enhance your bowel health or alleviate symptoms.

The Bovine Diet

Have you ever watched cattle in a field? You will notice that they spend a considerable amount of time grazing or eating small amounts of grass most of their waking day. If you were brought up in a farm community or ever walked in a pasture, you will note, if you just happened to have stepped in a cow paddy, that the pile of manure is formed and contains undigested grass and seeds. Now you know why there are little birds that will peck through cow dung, which provides the "hot lunch feeding program" for these tiny avians looking for undigested grains and other tasty nuggets. We can learn from our bovine friends the importance of grazing. For those who suffer from fecal incontinence, you should consider eating small, frequent meals, on the order of five to six a day instead of the customary three meals throughout the day. So be like a bovine and graze through smaller portions instead of consuming large quantities of food just a few times a day.

Certain food additives contribute to fecal incontinence, including sorbitol (found in artificial sweeteners), lactose, fructose, and excessive caffeine and alcohol. If your diet consists of large quantities of these substances, you will want to avoid or lessen them considerably. Lactose intolerance (i.e., inability to digest milk products), which is a result of a deficiency of an enzyme, lactase, is present in 25 percent of Americans and can result in gas, diarrhea, rectal urgency, and even fecal incontinence. When women completely avoid lactose, they have reported considerable improvement. However, if you love dairy products, taking over-the-counter lactase pills before your dairy meal can be helpful. Also, spicy, greasy foods and diet foods can exacerbate BCD. An excellent resource for women with fecal incontinence is the National Association For Continence (NAFC), www.nafc.org.

Foods and drinks that typically cause diarrhea, and so should probably be avoided, include the following:

- Drinks and foods containing caffeine
- Cured or smoked meat such as sausage, ham, or turkey
- Spicy foods
- Alcoholic beverages
- Dairy products such as milk, cheese, or ice cream
- Fruits such as apples, peaches, or pears
- Fatty and greasy foods
- Sweeteners, such as sorbitol, xylitol, mannitol, and fructose, which are found in diet drinks, sugarless gum and candy, chocolate, and fruit juices

---

Some women with BCD have experienced great improvement in their symptoms if they reduce the intake of insoluble fiber, which is found in whole-grain breads, cereals, nuts, beans, and corn. On the other hand, increasing the use of soluble fiber has been effective in reducing the episodes of fecal insentience. Sources of soluble fiber include bananas, rice, tapioca, bread, potatoes, applesauce, cheese, smooth peanut butter, yogurt, pasta, and oatmeal. These soluble foods tend to thicken, solidify, and increase caliber of your stools so that your rectum is more likely to sense the stool bolus and the anal sphincter is more likely to be able to keep it from leaking out. It is suggested that you need to eat 30 to 35 grams of fiber a day, but add it to your diet slowly so your body can adjust.

Overcoming Fecal Incontinence

Pelvic floor therapy for fecal incontinence consists of diet modification, biofeedback, and Kegel exercises. The purpose of pelvic floor therapy is to train the person to relearn how to control her bowel movements. Whether this will work for you depends on the cause of your fecal incontinence, how severe the muscle damage is, how well your rectum senses its contents, and your ability to do the exercises. If you have any questions, please consult with your doctor.

When Medicines and Surgery Are Recommended

When changing your diet does not help reduce your fecal incontinence, then you should consider medications. Certain medications can help treat fecal incontinence. Antibiotics are used to treat bacterial infections that cause diarrhea and fecal incontinence. Drugs are also effective to decrease the motility of the small and large intestines. One of the most commonly used drugs is loperamide (Lopex, Imodium, Dimor, Fortasec, and Pepto). Loperamide is also effective for increasing the pressure in the anal sphincter and thus prevent anal leakage. For patients with inflammatory bowel disease (Crohn's disease or ulcerative colitis), corticosteroids and immunosuppressant drugs can be used to decrease inflammation.

Irritable bowel syndrome (IBS) can also be alleviated by antispasmodic drugs, which may also help to decrease the tension in the colon and alleviate pain and bloating. For example, dicyclomine (Bentyl) can relieve cramping and spasms. Desipramine (Norpramin) is an antidepressant medication, which can also help with pain of IBS.

In 2008, a gastroenterologist from the University of Minnesota treated a patient with debilitating diarrhea and bowel control disorder as a result of *Clostridium difficile* (known as C-dif), a severe bacterial infection. The woman was on her deathbed and was wasting away from malnutrition due to her severe diarrhea. The treatment consisted of a fecal transplant when the doctor took bacteria from her husband and transplanted the good bacteria from her husband through an enema into the patient's colon. Within days after the transplant, the woman's diarrhea abated, the infection was gone, and her symptoms of bowel control disorder ceased.

In May 2011, the FDA approved Solesta, an injectable gel, for the treatment of fecal incontinence in patients who have failed other remedies. Solesta, a bulking agent, is injected just beneath the lining of the anus with the purpose of decreasing or narrowing the opening of the anus; this may help patients to better control their bowel movements.

One of the most common causes of vaginal pressure and rectal discomfort is a rectocele (described in Chapter Three), when there is a weakness in the vagina that allows the rectum to protrude through the vagina. This is to be differentiated from rectal prolapse, where the rectum protrudes out of the anus; rectal prolapse is another cause of fecal incontinence. The good news is that both of these conditions can be successfully repaired through a vaginal incision (for rectocele) or an anal incision (for rectal prolapse) in a one-day-stay surgical facility with recovery in just a few weeks (see Chapter Three).

Rectovaginal fistula, which is an abnormal communication from the anus and/or rectum to the vagina, is another condition that causes fecal incontinence. Usually, this condition is caused by childbirth injury, improper healing, infection, or Crohn's disease. A patient with this condition may complain of passing gas through her vagina or staining and leaking of liquid (and sometimes solid) stool through her vagina. Other conditions that can lead to rectovaginal fistula are infection of the anal glands, radiation, and cancer. Rectovaginal fistulae are usually treated by surgery. However, if the fistula is small, and the patient is not a good candidate for a fistula repair surgery, a fistula plug can be sewn into the hole during an outpatient procedure. This has a lower success rate than traditional surgery.

Tears of the anal sphincter can occur with vaginal deliveries and can result in loss of control of the anus. If an imaging study such as an ultrasound or MRI shows a significant tear in the anal sphincter and the patient still has good pudendal nerve function, then a sphincteroplasty is an option. A sphincteroplasty is a procedure used to reconstruct or repair the torn sphincter.

Secca™, a radiofrequency energy device, is another procedure for treatment of BCD. This procedure, which received FDA approval in

2002, may be effective for mild fecal incontinence and is performed in the operating room on an outpatient basis in less than 45 minutes. A device is inserted into the anus/rectum, and the internal anal sphincter is heated to 185 °F with the goal of tightening the anal canal.

In patients who have intact anal sphincter muscles but who have weak or no nerve function, neuromodulation may be a better option. Although the FDA has recently approved sacral neuromodulation (InterStim™) for treatment of fecal incontinence, it has been used successfully for many years in Europe. Recent studies suggest that InterStim may be better than anal sphincteroplasty for long-term treatment of fecal incontinence. (InterStim is discussed in more detail in Chapter Two).

When all else fails to control fecal incontinence, an ileostomy or colostomy can be created, which diverts the feces to the front of the lower abdomen. Although most colostomies are temporary when there are medical conditions affecting the colon, a permanent colostomy can be the last resort for the treatment of fecal incontinence. For temporary colostomies, when the condition has resolved with treatment, the colostomy can be closed, and normal defecation restored. It is important to have very good skin care to avoid irritation and infection of the skin around the opening or stoma on the front of the abdomen.

Now an artificial bowel sphincter is available as an implanted device that substitutes as the natural anal sphincter. This kind of option is suitable for young people who don't want to have a colostomy and who have been in a bad accident in which the anus was penetrated and nerves were damaged. The device, which consists of a cuff placed around the rectum, is attached to a reservoir inside the abdomen and a pump located in the outer lips, or labia major. When the device is active, the cuff compresses the rectum and holds the feces in the rectum.

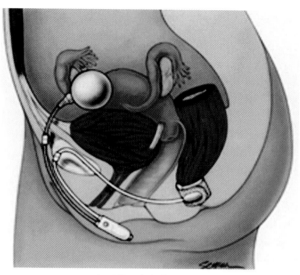

Artificial Sphincter

Testing Before Surgery

If conservative measures do not adequately relieve your BCD, then your doctor may consider surgery. Before any operation, he/she will perform tests in order to choose the best method of surgery for you. These important tests include an anal ultrasound or MRI, anal pressure measurements (or manometry), and nerve and muscle testing.

The Bottom Line

The bottom line is this: fecal incontinence is one of life's most miserable conditions that affect millions of American women. Most women can be helped with dietary modification, medication, or surgery in the most resistant cases. If you or someone you care about is suffering from this dreaded nuisance, please know help is on its way.

Suggestions to Control BCD

- Eat small meals more frequently. In some people, large meals cause bowel contractions that lead to diarrhea. You can still eat the same amount of food in a day, but space it out by eating several small meals.
- Eat and drink at different times. Liquid helps move food through the digestive system. So if you want to slow things down, drink something half an hour before or after meals, but not with meals.
- Eat the right amount of fiber. For many people, fiber makes stool soft, formed, and easier to control. Fiber is found in fruits, vegetables, and grains. You need to eat 30 to 35 grams of fiber a day, but add it to your diet slowly so your body can adjust. Too much fiber all at once can cause bloating, gas, or even diarrhea. Also, too much indigestible fiber can contribute to diarrhea. If you find that eating more fiber makes your diarrhea worse, try cutting back to two servings each of fruits and vegetables and removing skin and seeds from your food.

Down There Diet for Fecal Incontinence*

Eat foods that make stool bulkier. Foods that contain digestible fiber slow the emptying of the bowels, including bananas, rice, tapioca, bread, potatoes, applesauce, cheese, smooth peanut butter, yogurt, pasta, and oatmeal.

Get plenty to drink. Drink eight, 8 ounce glasses of liquid a day to help prevent dehydration and keep stool soft and formed. Water is a good choice. Avoid drinks with caffeine, alcohol, milk, or carbonation if you find they trigger diarrhea.

- Choose more fresh fruits and vegetables:
  apples
  pears
  bananas
  potatoes
  blueberries
  prunes
  broccoli
  raisins
  Brussels sprouts
  spinach
  cantaloupe
  strawberries
  carrots
  sweet potatoes
  figs
  tomatoes
  oranges
  zucchini
  peaches

- Choose more whole-grain breads, pastas, and cereals:
  All-Bran
  oat bran

barley
oatmeal
Bran Flakes
pumpernickel bread
brown rice
raisin bran
granola
whole-grain breads

- Choose more dried beans, peas, nuts, and
  seeds (as tolerated):
  baked beans
  split peas
  lentils
  sunflower seeds
  peanuts-walnuts
  soy products, such as tofu and textured vegetable protein

- Choose more snacks that are high in fiber:
  cereal mix with nuts and seeds
  fresh fruit
  fresh vegetables
  popcorn
  whole-grain cereal
  yogurt with bran cereal

- Plan more vegetarian meals:
  bean and rice burritos
  beans and rice
  hummus and pita bread
  pasta with vegetables
  split pea or lentil soup
  vegetable stir fry

*Modified from Urology Center of Columbus, LLC (http://www. harperurology.com/documentlibrary/115_Fecal%20 Incontinence.pdf).

Chapter Eight

When It's No Longer Fun Down There: Female Sexual Dysfunction

Barbara is a 52-year-old woman who has had lack of interest in sex for several years. She does not have sexual thoughts or fantasies anymore but does continue to have intercourse with her husband anyway. She uses a lubricant for vaginal dryness, and this does reduce her pain during intercourse. With proper stimulation, she can achieve orgasm. Although she is not concerned about her reduced libido, her husband is bothered by it. Despite his arthritis and high blood pressure, he does not have any problems with erection and has desire to have intercourse. Even though Barbara doesn't have any medical problems, she "just doesn't want to have sex anymore." As she says, "I feel like I am just going through the motions."

When asked if she thinks she may have desire disorder, Barbara responds, "My husband and I have an average relationship for our age." They have been married for almost 25 years, and she feels she is "as close to [her] husband as anyone can be after being married that long."

Barbara is one of the millions of women who silently, unwittingly accepts life with no sexual desire. Very likely, Barbara also has vaginal atrophy and would benefit from some local estrogen, but even more importantly, this couple would benefit from marital or couples counseling to make both partners more aware of what they can do to resuscitate their intimacy and realize that they do, in fact, have options to revive their mutual desire and satisfaction in sex.

But not all issues with sexual functioning strike women in perimenopause or menopause. Jennifer is a 29-year-old woman who came to see one of us because of loss of libido and is inquiring whether either hormones or Viagra would help with her low desire to have sex. She says that she has not had any sexual thoughts or fantasies for almost a year. She is married, is healthy, and has a healthy daughter who she delivered by normal vaginal childbirth four years ago. She does have intercourse with her partner to keep the peace, but their sexual encounters occur once or twice every two months. When they do have intercourse, they are both able to orgasm, but it now takes her a longer time to orgasm than it did when they first got married.

Jennifer says that she loves her husband but doesn't feel they are as close as they used to be when they first were married. He has a high-stress job and works more than 80 hours per week. When they do have time together, he is exhausted, and she is not interested in sex.

What is happening in this relationship? Most likely, there is nothing really wrong with Jennifer physically; rather, the lack of intimate time the couple spends together is undermining lack of sexual excitement, her sexual desire, and responsiveness. Very likely, since this couple doesn't spend enough time together, there is a lack of emotional closeness and tenderness, which, in turn, affects Jennifer's sense of well-being and happiness.

Unfortunately, Barbara and Jennifer are two of the millions of American women who suffer from female sexual dysfunction (FSD). Typically, this condition is associated with loss of desire for sexual intimacy or lack of arousal. Women usually also experience a lack of lubrication of the vagina. These symptoms are not only life-altering, but they can also lead to emotional distress and depression, and often get in the way of intimacy in even the strongest relationships.

But even more concerning to us is the emotional and social fallout from FSD: women feel so much shame regarding their symptoms and receive so little support or suggestions for treatment from their healthcare providers that literally millions of women suffer in silence, cutting themselves off from one of their most robust sources of pleasure and vitality. Indeed, a woman can experience her sensual self well into her eighties, despite the hormonal and other physiological shifts that occur after menopause.

Let's set the record straight. You are not alone. It is estimated that 63 percent of women (and 52 percent of men) suffer from some form of sexual dysfunction. In fact, 75 percent of couples who seek marital therapy report sexual concerns, and nearly 15 percent of married women have difficulty with intercourse and a similar percentage have painful intercourse leading to avoidance of intimacy all together. An even larger number of women fail to have an orgasm some or even all of the time. Now get ready for this statistic because it's alarming: nearly 75 percent of women have sexual dissatisfaction but are not classified as dysfunctional. This means that nearly all women have some element of sexual dissatisfaction or sexual dysfunction. If that wasn't alarming enough, one type of sexual dysfunction often triggers another type sexual dysfunction. For instance, a woman who might start with a seemingly bothersome problem of diminished orgasm can over time develop a much more entrenched problem with decreased desire, causing her to avoid sexual intimacy altogether.

Some women have a lifelong history of sexual dysfunction. Others develop sexual problems much later in life after having very normal sexual experiences as a younger woman. Take for example, Courtney, a 26-year-old woman who has been married for eight months. Prior to her wedding, she had only one boyfriend and never had sexual intercourse until her honeymoon. But since that time, she has become increasingly worried because although she is very attracted toward her husband and wants to have sex with him, she has never had an orgasm. She does not experience any pain with intercourse, has no history of abuse, and has no health problems. She and her husband are very close and have a loving relationship, and they have intercourse three times a week.

Why can't Courtney have an orgasm? This is a good example of orgasmic dysfunction that is most common in young, less experienced women. Courtney would benefit from seeing a sex therapist for sex education and sensate focus therapy and learn more about how her body works. She would benefit from learning how to masturbate on her own first so she can orgasm and then communicate the experience to her husband. She might also benefit from, and enjoy, mutual masturbation.

In another case, Laura, who is 35 years old, came to see us complaining of severe pelvic pain (chronic pelvic pain, or CPP). For the last six years, she has also experienced excruciating pain, or dyspareunia, every time she attempts to have intercourse. In the past, when she is about to be intimate with her partner, she suddenly feels an almost uncontrollable urge to push him away, and her thighs automatically clench around him; this involuntary reaction is known as vaginismus. On occasions, even partial penetration of her vagina causes her pain so unbearable that she cannot help but to cry uncontrollably.

Because Laura has experienced these symptoms for most of her adult, dating life, she has lost several boyfriends because of this. As a result, she had been avoiding forming intimate relationships. She has seen several doctors and spent lots of money and was told that her external and internal reproductive organs are normal and that all the lab tests have been normal as well. She was told by one doctor that it "is all in your head." Another told her that "you have recurrent yeast infections." One of the doctors she had seen told her that her pelvic muscles were very firm and tender almost like someone who has cramping in their legs after sprinting. Her medical history is unremarkable, but after extensive interviewing, she does admit to being sexually abused as a child.

History of sexual abuse is uncovered in up to 50 percent of patients with CPP and with dyspareunia (i.e., the above scenario). The best treatment for her is to see a psychologist. After a period of intensive psychotherapy, she would also benefit from seeing a sex therapist and will need to use vaginal dilators to help her with her vaginismus.

The good news is that there is a much greater understanding of female sexual functioning, physiology, and malfunctioning of the organs located down there. In addition, effective options for women with FSD are now available so that for proactive women who seek treatment, most can refind their sexual self again and the pleasure and fun that comes with it.

Let's take a look at what conditions actually qualify as FSD so that you can determine whether or not you have one or more symptoms and what you can do about them.

The Most Common FSDs

Doctors have been trying for years to get their arms around FSD, trying to categorize all of the issues so that they can provide treatment options that really work. The global definition of FSD refers to "a lack of enjoyment with sexual intimacy with your partner." However, there are categories of FSD that are helpful for arriving at a diagnosis and, ultimately, at a treatment to successfully resolve this cluster of problems. We would like for you to think of FSD in the following four categories: desire disorders, orgasmic difficulties, arousal disorders, and pain disorders.

The most common FSDs include the following:

- Hypoactive sexual desire disorder—This condition is indicated by a loss of desire for sex and affects up to 26 percent of women resulting in the loss in sexual yearning or fantasizing. When the desire is diminished or lost, there can be significant conflict and tension between the partners. Nothing can lead to marital discord faster than a woman who has lost her interest and a man who has fire in his loins.
- Female sexual arousal disorder—This FSD is a disruption in a woman's ability to become physically aroused and is most clearly marked by a lack of vaginal lubrication.
- Female orgasmic disorder—This is an inability to reach orgasm (or a diminished intensity in orgasm) from either self-stimulation or during sexual intimacy with a partner, or both; an orgasmic disorder often coexists with arousal disorder.
- Dyspareunia—This is the experience of intense or severe pain from penetration during intercourse.
- Vaginismus—This condition is marked by a tightening of the muscles in the pelvis, making penetration during intercourse difficult or impossible; vaginismus is often associated with or caused by a fear of vaginal penetration.
- Vulvodynia—This is a condition of chronic pain around the opening of the vagina (or vulva) for which there is no identifiable cause (see Chapter Five for further details).

How FSDs Are Different from Other Issues Down There

It was Drs. William H. Masters and Virginia Johnson who in 1966 first made an effort to scientifically study male and female sexual responses. They describe four phases for both men and women: excitement, plateau, orgasmic, and resolution phases. By inserting small cameras into the vaginas of women, they were able to study the sexual responses of hundreds of normal women. It is our guess that they didn't have to wait long for "volunteers" to appear for this interesting research! Their research found that during excitement phases, the clitoris and the labia minora become engorged with blood, and there is marked increase in the length of the vagina and the clitoris. They observed that the size of the labia minora increase during sexual excitement, and there is a blossoming of the labia, thus exposing their inner surface.

The current classification of FSD presents a more nonlinear view of how women experience desire, become aroused, respond to sexual excitement, and reach orgasm. This new model for understanding how women's sexual functioning works integrates emotional intimacy, sexual stimuli, and relationship satisfaction, and underscores the difficulty distinguishing between desire and arousal. For some women, desire does not always precede arousal; for other women, desire has to be present in order to become sexually aroused.

For this reason, causes of FSD can be complicated. The lines between the physical (often hormonal), psychological, and emotional causes frequently overlap, making it difficult for both women and their doctors to tease out the exact causes for a woman's condition. Most FSD is caused by a combination of physical and psychological factors. For example, a woman can have a physical reason why she has difficulty having intercourse. If the physical discomfort persists over time, there is likelihood that emotional and psychological causes will also emerge thus making the problem worse. As a result, there is a great overlap among the FSDs. It is not possible to single out one entity that is responsible for the FSD. That is why you need to seek out a physician who understands these ramifications and treats the whole patient both emotionally and physically.

Sandra is 40 years of age and has had painful intercourse for nearly five years. As a result, she makes every effort to avoid intimacy with her partner because she knows that the experience is anything but enjoyable. Her partner is understanding, but she knows full well that his level of frustration is reaching the boiling point. There is constant bickering and arguing over issues that wouldn't have resulted in any discord a few years ago. She complained to her physician that she and her family noted that she was less energetic and decreasing her interaction with her friends and family. She sought out treatment from her primary care doctor, who did not take a sexual history, and diagnosed her with depression. He started her on antidepressant medication, which did improve her mood but did absolutely nothing for sexual dysfunction. It wasn't until she consulted with her gynecologist that the sexual history was taken and the painful intercourse was addressed and resolved. Sandra was then able to return to sexual activity, and both she and her husband became happy campers.

How Your Hormonal Life Cycle Can Interfere

The physical causes of FSD are usually related to changes in the hormonal balance that often accompanies menopause. The two female hormones estrogen and progesterone, which are both produced in the ovaries, have an enormous role in a woman's metabolism, well-being, and sexual functioning. When these hormones are present and working together in a coordinated fashion, a woman's metabolism, mental status, and ability to engage in sexual intimacy with enjoyment and pleasure have a much higher likelihood of working in harmony. However, once a woman is in perimenopause, defined as the menopausal transition or the interval in which a woman's body makes a natural shift from more or less regular cycles of ovulation and menstruation toward permanent infertility, or menopause, she can experience a natural deficiency in one or both of these hormones, triggering loss of lubrication and lessening of desire and responsiveness. Perimenopause is most common when a woman is in her late forties, or rarely even as early as her thirties. Most of these deficiencies occur when a woman enters menopause, which is on average around age 51, but can also occur in younger or older women. Indeed, women in their thirties and forties can also experience drops in their estrogen levels during their menstrual cycle, causing vaginal dryness to occur.

In addition to estrogen and progesterone, testosterone, the main hormone in men, also has an important role in a woman's sex drive, libido, and overall interest in engaging in sexual activities. Testosterone, which is also produced in the ovary and smaller amounts in the adrenal gland (a small endocrine gland that is located on the top of each kidney), does effectively boost sex drive—as well as remedy other sexual problems.

Testosterone is known as the personality hormone. It gives us motivation, assertiveness, a sense of power, a feeling of well-being, and enhanced sex drive. When we have adequate levels of testosterone, we are able to take risks and live our lives with zest. Without testosterone, we exist as if in black and white. It is testosterone that brings us into full living color. Testosterone conveys powerful antiaging effects. It turns fat into muscle, keeps skin supple, increases bone mineral density, gives us positive mood, and boosts our ability to handle stress. It supports cognitive functioning and keeps the liver and blood vessels clean. Low-testosterone levels have been associated with heart attack, Alzheimer's disease, osteoporosis, and depression. At the time of menopause, the ovaries become less efficient, and the hormone levels of estrogen, progesterone, and testosterone begin to decrease. Eventually, the ovaries stop making estrogen and progesterone altogether, and the vaginal walls become drier, thinner, and less elastic, which, when left untreated, can make intercourse painful.

Just as one of the main causes affecting a man's ability to have an erection is a decrease in the blood supply to the penis, women are also affected by conditions that narrow the opening of the blood vessels that supply the vagina and clitoris. Consequently, nutrients and oxygen are less plentiful, and there are changes that take place in the vagina resulting in loss of the normal elastic tissue, increase in firm fibrous tissue formation, and loss of lubrication at the time of sexual arousal. These vascular changes also affect the nerve endings in the clitoris. So it is not surprising that these changes also result in loss of sensation making it more difficult for the woman to achieve an orgasm. One of our colleagues, Dr. Irwin Goldstein, who is a national expert on FSD, refers to this scenario as "heart attack of the vagina." Just as a decrease in blood supply to the heart results in decrease oxygen to the heart muscle and causes chest pain, a lack of blood supply to the pelvis is also problematic for sexual arousal. All these factors mean women often have pain and discomfort at the time of sexual intimacy. As a result, the woman finds reasons to defer intimacy because she wants to avoid pain and soreness after having intercourse.

However, the pain, lack of lubrication, and loss of libido associated with FSD are often avoidable and easily treatable, resulting in significant improvement in your ability to enjoy sexual intimacy once again. Indeed, we believe that there is a myth circulating even in the medical literature that aging results in sexual dysfunction in both men and women. Nothing could be further from the truth. As a matter of fact, it is common for older, menopausal women to be able to engage and enjoy sexual intimacy as they get older. They may need some assistance with estrogen and vaginal lubrication, but what a small price to pay for being able to be sexually intimate with the one they love.

Medical Causes of Problems Down There

Drugs

Although medications can be helpful and beneficial for those who need them, they also are associated with side effects or adverse effects that can impact a woman's sexual functioning. Even contraceptives may result in a decrease in estrogen level, vaginal dryness and loss in libido. An oral contraceptive with a high ratio of estrogen to progestin may resolve that problem.

In addition to hormonal contraceptives, a surprising number of drugs can interfere with sexual functioning. These include the following:

- Antidepressants, including selective serotonin reuptake inhibitors (SSRIs), such as fluoxetine (Prozac) and paroxetine (Paxil), can alter brain chemicals that affect sexual desire and response.
- Antibiotics, especially if used for a long period of time, can cause yeast infections, making intercourse uncomfortable.
- Antihistamines dry all mucous membranes including those of the vagina.
- Heart and blood pressure medicines cause sexual dysfunction in many of women taking them. Some of the these medications can lower the desire for sexual intimacy
- Tranquilizers can lower libido and delay or prevent orgasm.
- Diet aids, sleep aids, and other over-the-counter drugs can cause drowsiness, reduce sexual desire, cause dryness, and impair function.
- Chemotherapy with toxic drugs can cause fatigue and nausea and result in a decreased sex drive.
- Alcohol, smoking, and illicit drugs may impair sexual function.

(A summary of these medications causing FSD is listed at the end of this chapter.)

Infections

If a woman has a urinary tract infection (UTI), a vaginal infection, or a sexually transmitted disease (STD), she may have difficulty with sexual intimacy and can have pain with intercourse. On the other hand, it is not uncommon for women to take antibiotics for these infections and then develop a yeast infection that causes vaginal discharge and rawness around the vagina making intimacy difficult or impossible. You may find that daily yogurt containing *Lactobacillus acidophilus* bacteria can help prevent these yeast infections.

Medical Illnesses

Nearly any medical problem affecting the endocrine glands, such as too much or too little thyroid hormone or an adrenal gland problem, can result in sexual dysfunction.

Two of the most common medical conditions associated with FSD are diabetes and atherosclerosis or narrowing of the blood vessels from cholesterol deposits into the blood vessel lining. Both diabetes and atherosclerosis are accompanied by a decrease in the blood flow to the vagina and clitoris, resulting in a decrease in lubrication and a decrease in sensitivity of the clitoris leading to decrease in pleasure and difficulty achieving an orgasm.

Pelvic Surgery

Extensive surgical procedures for cancers of the ovary, bladder, rectum, and uterus can result in early menopause, as can chemotherapy for breast cancer. Many of these surgical procedures are accompanied by radiation to the pelvis. This too can affect the nerves and blood vessels resulting in decreased sensation and loss of lubrication in the vagina during sexual arousal.

Surgery for prolapse, especially if *vaginal* mesh was used, can result in exposure, contraction, and stiffness of the mesh and vagina; this can lead to pain for both the woman and her partner (if mesh is exposure). See Chapter Three for more detail.

Although breast surgery doesn't take place down there, the women who have had mastectomies for breast cancer often have FSD. Many women who have had breast cancer surgery will not have sexual intimacy for many months after they leave the hospital. After breast cancer and mastectomy, many women will never use the female on top position during sexual intimacy. These women also have a significant decrease in enjoyment from breast stimulation. Also, many of the partners of women who have had breast surgery are either afraid to touch or look at their partner's mastectomy scar for several months after the operation. For this reason, it is quite common—and understandable—that women with breast cancer can develop feelings of decreased femininity, loss of self-esteem, a distortion of self-image, a sense of body disfigurement, and the untoward affect of chemotherapy on libido, arousal, and decrease in vaginal lubrication.

Injuries and Hysterectomy

Pelvic fractures can result in a disruption of the blood and nerve supply to the vagina and clitoris resulting in a loss of sensation and problems achieving an orgasm. Spinal cord injuries can affect sensation to and from the vagina and clitoris making sexual functioning difficult but not impossible.

Gynecologic conditions such as endometriosis, fibroids, infections of the uterus or fallopian tubes, prolapse, and incontinence can have a significant impact on sexual functioning.

It is of interest that a hysterectomy often has a beneficial effect on sexual function especially if the ovaries are left intact. Many women will report that when the pain, discomfort, and vaginal bleeding is gone, they are able to have a more enjoyable sex life. Also, the fear of pregnancy is gone after a hysterectomy, and the couple no longer has to be anxious about an unwanted pregnancy. Dr. Domeena Renshaw, one of the foremost sex therapists from Chicago's Stritch School of Medicine, reminds us that it isn't the uterus that is responsible for arousal, it is the clitoris as well as that organ between woman's ears—her brain!

The Emotional and Mental Roots of FSD

FSD does not happen in a vacuum. Seldom do women with FSD have an isolated problem without any psychological manifestations. It is part of the Venus makeup of women to be sexual and to enjoy intimacy with their partner. When this is removed or diminished, psychological manifestations are likely to accompany FSD. As a result, treating only one component such as the emotional problem with antidepressants will not resolve the total problem. This is just one more reason that we suggest that you receive care from a doctor who understands FSD and its psychological ramifications.

There is probably no bodily function that combines the interaction of the mind-body connection than a woman's sexuality. Any emotional or psychological problem can be a primary cause of a woman's FSD and also be a contributing factor if there are concomitant medical problems or if the woman uses one or more medications. Even if a woman does not have a diagnosed mental condition, emotional problems can result in FSD. Examples of psychological causes of FSD include stress and fatigue. Women, who are distracted and under significant stress, may have a decrease in desire and not be interested in sexual intimacy.

Sandra is a 40-year-old woman who is caring for a chronically sick child with Crohn's disease and also taking care of her elderly parents, who have moved into her home. She truly understands the concept of the sandwich generation that so many middle-aged women have joined. Sandra was previously orgasmic and enjoyed and looked forward to participating in sexual intimacy with her husband. However, with added burden of her parents in her home, there has been a significant loss of sexual intimacy accompanied by a decrease in her libido and her interest in sexual activity. Her gynecologist referred her and her husband to a counselor, and with a short course of couples therapy and antidepressants for Sandra, the couple have regained their enjoyment in sexual intimacy.

The same situation of emotional impact on a woman's sexual appetite also applies to significant fatigue where lack of sleep can result in a decrease or total absence of libido until a more restful state is achieved. Many women today who are faced with balancing a career and family are working 16 to 18 hours a day. Is it any wonder that these women prefer going to sleep than making love to their partner?

Jane and her husband have been married for seven years. Jane is a 30-year-old lawyer who works for a prestigious law firm. Her husband is three years older and is a mechanic and works nine to five. For the last year, they have been trying to have a baby but have been unsuccessful. After seeing their gynecologist, they were told that everything is in order biologically, but that they need to have intercourse more often. Jane is trying to make partner at the law firm and has been putting in 16 hours a day including most weekends. She is usually too tired to have sex and falls asleep before her husband comes into bed. Her husband says that on occasion during a weekend when his wife does have energy she is so preoccupied with her work that sex is the very last thing on her mind.

Another psychological cause is poor communication with the woman's partner. Sexual intimacy requires more than vaginal penetration. It requires open avenues of communication between the partners. If communication is lacking, there will be a conflicted or nonexistent sex life. Communication problems, anger, a lack of trust, a lack of connection, and a lack of intimacy can all adversely affect a woman's sexual interest and receptivity for engaging in sexual intimacy. If a woman doesn't trust the faithfulness of her partner, sexual intimacy will not be easy, and the likelihood of a decrease in libido, arousal, and lubrication may occur.

Unrealistic expectations by one or both partners can result in an unfilled sexual relationship.

Religious inhibitions can also affect a woman's sexual functioning in later life. If a woman is a member of a religious organization that looks negatively at premarital sex or self-stimulation, there may be feelings of guilt associated with intimacy that decrease her libido and her ability to be aroused. Vaginismus can also be manifested in women who have strict religious upbringing.

Legacy of Abuse

Women who have had the unfortunate experience of sexual or emotional abuse as children are very likely to experience sexual dysfunction as adults. Women who have been sexually or emotionally abused in childhood or adolescence often face a range of sexual difficulties. They may experience involuntary muscle tightening down there, making penetration impossible or very painful (vaginismus). On the other extreme, some women become overtly promiscuous pursuing multiple sexual encounters in ways that ultimately harm their self-esteem and sense of self. Some women may develop sex addiction and require intensive psychotherapy and other forms of intervention to control their self-sabotaging behavior.

Numerous psychological causes can result in negative impact on a woman's sexual performance. For example, depression is a disease that is more common in women than in men and results in loss of all appetites including the appetite for sexual intimacy. In addition, the treatment for depression using antidepressants such as SSRIs like fluoxetine and paroxetine can negatively impact libido and arousal, which compounds the problem of women suffering from depression.

Self-esteem plays an important role in a woman's sexual function. It is not surprising that women today can suffer from an altered body image and a diminished self-esteem. If you look at any fashion magazine, you will note quickly that these publications promote such unrealistic images of beauty that only very small number of women can live up to. Women with a decreased self-esteem, such as after a mastectomy, will be the ones who turn out the lights during sex, and sometimes even while undressing. If a woman doesn't feel good about her body or herself, or doesn't feel as in control or powerful, it's extremely hard for her to let go and sexually respond to her partner.

Fears Related to Female Sexual Dysfunction

Women are also prone to develop sexual dysfunction after childbirth. Sex may feel different after childbirth. Some women may experience pain as a result of abnormal healing of a tear in the vagina and perineum as a result of the baby's head stretching the vaginal opening. The added stress and exhaustion of taking care of a new baby, the change in the dynamics of relationship with her partner after a new family member is added, along with postpartum blues often can lead to reduced interest in sex. Breastfeeding also keeps estrogen at low levels. All these internal and external pressures contribute to sexual dysfunction in some women after childbirth.

If a woman is fearful about becoming pregnant or getting an STD she won't be able to relax and enjoy sexual intimacy. That's one reason why women who have a hysterectomy are able to be more relaxed during sex as they no longer have fear of becoming pregnant.

Women with urinary incontinence (see Chapter Two) will frequently have FSD. A woman with coital incontinence not only may become a spectator during sexual intercourse because of fear of loss of control of her bladder, but she also may be embarrassed and fearful of sexual intimacy altogether. Over time, this may lead to desire not to have sex, and this can in turn affect the marriage. Treatment of the incontinence will often resolve this FSD.

Another group of women who are at risk for FSD are those who have lost a partner and have not engaged in sexual intimacy for several years. These women are often postmenopausal and suffer from estrogen deficiency and have thinned out vaginal lining (vaginal atrophy). In addition, the vaginal opening has become constricted, making vaginal penetration painful or impossible. As a result, women in this situation are fearful of entering into a sexual relationship because of the anticipated pain and discomfort that they fear will accompany vaginal penetration. It's very important that if you find yourself in this situation to seek out care from your doctor who can offer you immediate therapy.

Getting the Help You Need

If you are experiencing some of the symptoms of FSD and are fearful about visiting a doctor, you are not alone. Most women suffer in silence as they are embarrassed to ask their primary care doctor or their gynecologist about their sexual problems. As Sharon said, "Just thinking about the pain I experience makes me feel inadequate in some way. I always felt my doctor would think less of me if I brought up the subject" or "I don't think my doctor will understand and won't take me seriously."

To our minds, these misgivings about asking for help and being direct with your doctor about FSD underscore the delicacy of these conditions. We want you to rest assured that there are caring, knowledgeable, and responsive doctors and practitioners who are there to help you! Here are some steps to take so you can take care of yourself and put your sex life back on track and where you would like it to be.

First, try to determine if you have an FSD. Ask yourself these questions:

1. Do I have a decreased libido or a lack of sex drive?
2. Do I have difficulty becoming aroused and do I have decreased lubrication when I am aroused?
3. Am I unable or do I have difficulty having an orgasm on a consistent basis?
4. Do I have pain during intercourse or vaginal contact?

If you answered yes to one or more of these questions, you may have an FSD and can be helped if you seek treatment with a doctor who is knowledgeable about the problems that are associated with FSD. On the other hand, if you have any or all of the above symptoms but you and your partner are not bothered by them and they are not affecting your quality of life, then you do not have FSD and no treatment is required.

The very good news is that there are multiple ways you can get help for your FSD. In the past, very little could be done for the treatment of women who had lost the pleasure and fun down there. But now researchers, doctors, and some very savvy sex educators have developed multiple approaches to addressing issues of desire and libido, sexual functioning and responsiveness, as well as the pain and emotional issues that come with FSD. Before looking at the medical interventions, let's review what you can do on your own.

Nonmedical Treatments

If you are suffering from a decrease in lubrication, you can find an easy solution in a tube of K-Y Jelly™, Astroglide™, or other safe lubricants. A small amount of a lubricant, about the amount of toothpaste you would place on your toothbrush, before or during sexual foreplay will easily and quickly overcome dryness. Women may find that they can reach an orgasm more easily without the pressure of pleasing their partner and in privacy when masturbating or using a vibrator. We recommend Lelo personal massagers, They are elegantly designed massagers from Sweden that help women reduce stress, strengthen the pelvic floor muscles, and develop and fortify their core. These are massagers for those who enjoy having intense pleasure at their fingertips. They are available at Lelo.com.

A woman who has difficulty achieving orgasm during sex with her partner may find that she can achieve an orgasm through self-stimulation.

For women who have difficulty having an orgasm even with masturbation, some extra stimulation with a vibrator before having sex with your partner, may be helpful. You might need rubbing or stimulation for up to an hour before having sex. If you want orgasm with intercourse, you or your partner may want to gently stroke your clitoris. Women in this situation have to experiment and find their hot buttons and make sure those buttons are pushed either by themselves or by their partner.

Arousal disorder can also be improved with the use of Eros therapy. This device is a small handheld medical device that uses a gentle vacuum to improve your sexual responses by increasing blood flow to the clitoris and external genitalia. It is lightweight, easy to use, FDA approved, and available by a doctor's prescription only. The Eros device is used in the privacy of your home and should be used three to four times per week to achieve the maximum benefits. You may use the Eros device either prior to having intercourse or therapeutically without having intercourse. The device serves as a conditioning routine to restore blood flow to your clitoris and genitalia and to increase orgasms, vaginal lubrication, and your overall sexual satisfaction (cost is $395 and available at www.eros-therapy.com).

For women who have severe pain associated with vaginal penetration, or vaginismus, they can be helped with gentle, progressive vaginal dilatation. This consists of the use of commercial dilators or tampons of increasing size that are lubricated and then placed into the vagina for 15 minutes twice a day. Once the woman can easily accept a dilator, which is the same size as her partner's penis, then vaginal penetration by the partner can be tried. Using this incremental approach, nearly all women with vaginismus can be treated.

For women who are experiencing problems with arousal or decreasing libido, it's important that they look at certain lifestyle habits that may be causing or exacerbating the symptoms. Excessive alcohol consumption and drugs of abuse, such as cocaine and marijuana, are linked to decreases in desire and arousal. As the great bard, William Shakespeare once said about alcohol, "It provokes the desire, but it takes away the performance." Those immortal words still ring true today. Alcohol generally makes women and men more willing to have sex but less capable of the act. Alcohol reduces sexual arousal in women as well as men. Alcohol can reduce vaginal lubrication by reducing the blood flow to the vagina and clitoris. In moderate to large quantities, alcohol can make orgasm difficult to achieve. There have been many a man who was excited about the possibility of intimacy with his partner after a wonderful dinner including several bottles of champagne only to find that his amour went to sleep as soon as she lay down on her bed. So take a good look at your alcohol consumption, and if you notice that the desire is decreased after imbibing more than two glasses of wine or champagne, then consider reducing your alcohol intake or dilute the alcohol you do consume. Can you say, "Make mine a wine spritzer?"

Smoking is also a no-no. The active ingredient in cigarettes, nicotine, can restrict the blood supply to the pelvic tissues, especially the clitoris and vulva. Thus, the arousal as well as vaginal lubrication may be decreased. So if you are a cigarette smoker, this is one more reason for you to consider kicking the habit. Just think about the warning on cigarettes as "Cigarette Smoking May be Hazardous to Your Sexual Health!"

Supplements that Can Help FSD

The supplement DHEA (dehydroepiandrosterone) is a hormone produced naturally by the adrenal glands and is then converted to estrogen and testosterone; as you age, your body converts less and less of DHEA into sex hormones. But DHEA supplements have been shown to increase both estrogen and testosterone levels and have been helpful in postmenopausal women with decreased sexual desire or decreased libido. Side effects that have been reported include acne, male pattern hair growth, weight gain around the waist, high blood pressure, and decreased levels of HDL, or good, cholesterol.

Ginko biloba is an herb used for centuries in traditional Chinese medicine as a remedy for respiratory conditions, cognitive impairment, and circulatory disorders. Ginkgo may also help women with sexual dysfunction related to mood disorders.

L-arginine is an amino acid that has numerous functions in the body—especially to make nitric oxide, a compound that helps to relax blood vessels and allow blood to flow through arteries and carry oxygen and nutrients to the tissues. As a result, if there is a decrease in arousal and a decrease in lubrication, L-arginine, in large quantities, can dilate blood vessels and may increase the blood supply to the genital area as well. Food sources that are rich in L-arginine include plant and animal proteins, such as dairy products, meat, poultry, fish, soy, and nuts help direct more blood to the genitals, which means more lubrication and may help with arousal difficulties.

These natural remedies may help you correct your FSD. For women who experience one or more symptoms, or whose FSD seems related to a combination of factors both physical and emotional, or who have two or more physical symptoms at the same time (arousal and libido, for instance, or dyspareunia and anorgasmia), we recommend scheduling an appointment with your doctor to discuss these issues.

Hormones to the Rescue

Estrogen

The mainstay of treatment for arousal disorders or lack of lubrication is estrogen therapy. Estrogen replacement therapy is indicated for menopausal women (women in their fifties, sixties, or older) who may be estrogen deficient. It is common for arousal disorders to accompany natural menopause (see Chapter Nine), and arousal disorder can also occur in younger women who have had surgical menopause (i.e., if both ovaries are removed before they have gone through natural menopause). Estrogen supplements can be supplied with oral tablets, skin patches containing estrogens, topical vaginal creams, sprays, or estrogen rings that are inserted into the vagina. Oral estrogen and estrogen patches are both helpful for the symptoms of menopause, including hot flashes and preventing osteoporosis, or loss of bone density (see Chapter Nine on menopause).

Topical estrogens that are available as estrogen creams and an estrogen ring are helpful for restoring sensitivity of the clitoris, increasing vaginal lubrication, decreasing vaginal burning, decreasing the pain associated with sexual intimacy, and reducing urinary frequency.

The vaginal walls contain an abundance of tissues that contain estrogen receptors and are thus very sensitive to estrogen. A lack of estrogen results in atrophy of the vaginal lining, which becomes pale, thin, and dry and does not secrete the juices necessary to reduce the friction associated with intercourse. Topical estrogen creams or an estrogen ring placed in the vagina can easily solve this problem. Often postmenopausal women who use oral estrogens for reducing the symptoms of menopause may require supplemental topical estrogens to restore the vaginal lining toward normal and also to increase the lubrication at the time of sexual arousal. Women who still have their uterus and who use daily topical estrogens will also require supplemental progesterone in order to prevent problems of the lining of the uterus (also see Chapter Nine). Because of its low potency, the estrogen ring is usually not associated with absorption of estrogen from the vagina, and there is no need for supplemental progesterone.

Testosterone Therapy for Women Too?

Yes, that's right and not a misprint. Testosterone is also part of a woman's physiologic makeup and a necessary requirement for maintaining sexual interest and libido. Until very recently, it was not known what role testosterone played in women's metabolism and particularly in their sexual functioning. Now we know that it has a major role. You don't want to leave home without it!

A deficiency of testosterone in women is easily detected by a measuring the testosterone level and a protein (called SHBG) in the blood. If it is diminished, testosterone replacement is easily accomplished. Daily oral testosterone, 0.25 to 1.25 mg of methyltestosterone, is helpful, and the dosage is usually adjusted based on the woman's response of improved libido and an increased desire for sexual intimacy. Testosterone is also available in a patch and a cream for vaginal use. Now there are pellets (Testopel) containing testosterone that can be inserted under the skin in the buttocks or in the hip area. These are long-acting sources of testosterone and will last for four to six months before another implant is required. The blood levels of testosterone should be monitored carefully. If the blood levels of testosterone are above normal levels for prolonged periods of time, there are potential side effects that will be discussed later.

For women with both decreased desire and decreased vaginal lubrication, a combination of testosterone and estrogen may be indicated. This is available in a pill form as Estratest. There is also a skin ointment that can be made by a special compounding pharmacist. This skin application of testosterone may have fewer side effects.

So what's the big deal? The benefits of testosterone therapy in women with FSD include improvement in desire for sexual intimacy, increased vaginal and clitoral sensitivity, increased vaginal lubrication, and heightened arousal.

However, there are some potential side effects of testosterone therapy that women should consider, including weight gain, enlargement of the clitoris, increase in facial hair, and elevation of the blood cholesterol level. There are rare instances of liver disease and breast cancer, but this has not been a significant detractor for using testosterone in those women who are in need of this hormone for treating their FSD. Testosterone can be helpful for women with low desire.

Women who have been treated for breast cancer, women with severe liver disease, or women who have an abnormally elevated cholesterol level are not candidates for testosterone replacement therapy.

Other Considerations

For women with pelvic pain associated with deep penile thrusting, your doctor will need to rule out pelvic diseases such as endometriosis (Chapter Five) or significant pelvic organ prolapse (Chapter Three), which can be treated with surgery and easily resolve the discomfort. On the other hand, sexual pain that develops only after having pelvic surgery should be evaluated by the type of specialists (eg. FPMRS or Female Urologist) discussed in Chapter One, and this too can be managed effectively.

Women using antidepressant medications sometimes experience some sexual dysfunction, which can be related to their SSRI antidepressants. If you think that medicine you are taking may be impacting your libido or sexual responsiveness, then you should see your doctor to discuss whether you have alternatives. If the antidepressant is the culprit, then switching to another type of antidepressant, adjusting to a lower dosage, or temporarily stopping the medication, often can remedy sexual dysfunction. For example, one antidepressant, bupropion (Wellbutrin) may have a beneficial effect on libido in premenopausal women without depression and with hypoactive sexual desire disorder. Approximately one-third of women with severe acquired global hypoactive sexual desire disorder reported an increase in various measures of libido while on three hundred milligram daily.

Viagra for Women?

"If it is good for the gander, it must be good for the goose [female]!" Viagra (sildenafil) was developed in 1998 to help men achieve and maintain erection adequate for vaginal penetration. Viagra has been tested in women and may increase the blood supply to the clitoris and may be helpful with problems associated with arousal, vaginal dryness, and SSRI use. The drug appears to be most beneficial in women with decreased arousal, and some women report that Viagra heightens stimulation and sensitivity. Some women who have used Viagra report increased sexual arousal, enhanced lubrication, and more intense orgasms. The dosage of Viagra for women is the same as the dosage for men, 25 to 100 mg 30 to 45 minutes before engaging in sexual intimacy. The drug should not be used under any circumstance in women who are using nitrates for heart disease.

Let's Talk About It

Sometimes, medication or surgery is not enough to help women overcome their sexual problem. Since FSD may have more than one cause and can certainly have psychological implications, you may want to consider talking with a counselor or therapist. We suggest that you seek out a counselor who specializes in sexual and relationship problems. Usually this counseling occurs with a sex therapist. A sex therapist is a specially trained mental health professional who can be a psychologist, psychiatrist, or a clinical social worker. The sex therapist works in collaboration with other healthcare professionals to address the individual's or couples' sexual problems. A sex therapist would be particularly helpful in situations of decreased desire, problems with arousal, lack of orgasm, and pelvic pain especially pain associated with intercourse. Sex therapy usually works best if both parties in the relationship attend the therapy sessions. Sex therapy consists of talking to couples about their sexual lives, and the therapist will not be embarrassed if you bring it up. The therapist is there to help the woman and her partner gain understanding of some of the relationship dynamics and background issues that may be influencing the problem. The therapist can also provide you with information about human sexuality and sexual functioning and answer your questions. Oftentimes a woman with FSD will see both a medical doctor and a therapist to deal with the physical causes as well as the psychological ones.

Sex therapy with a certified and qualified sex therapist can be very helpful if there are problems with communication between the partners. If a woman has coexisting psychological problems such as depression, a sex therapist or the doctor treating the woman for depression may be able to help with the sexual dysfunction as well. Sex therapy is generally short term (approximately three months in duration) and can be conducted in an individual, couples, or even in a group setting. Stanley Althof, PhD, a renowned sex therapist in West Palm Beach, Florida, states that individual therapy is recommended for women with lifelong sexual problems. However, if the sexual problem develops after a time of normal sexual functioning, then individual or couples therapy is an the option.

FSD is complicated and usually involves a combination of emotional and physical factors; opening avenues of communication between partners can perform wonders. It is important to let your partner know what you like and dislike so that he or she can give you more of the former and avoid the latter. If verbalizing your likes and dislikes is difficult, consider writing each other a letter and then exchanging letters followed by a discussion.

According to Dr. Althof, approximately two-thirds of women who complete a course of sex therapy report significant improvements in their sex life. Over time, the gains may diminish. This is normal, and a woman may need to return to the therapist for a few booster sessions to help overcome backsliding into old negative patterns.

The American Association for Marriage and Family Therapy (AAMFT) has a therapist locater on its website (http://www.aamft.org/) to help you find a therapist in your area. There are two organizations that credential sex therapists. These are the Society for Sex Therapy and Research (http://www.sstarnet.org/) and American Association of Sexuality Educators, Counselors, and Therapists (http://www.aasect.org). Both of these organizations have a Find a Professional section that lists certified sex therapist in each state.

The Bottom Line

So what's the bottom line on FSD and the treatment of FSD? We have never seen happier patients than those women who have had FSD and found a successful resolution to their problem. These women report a significant reduction in stress, they have a better night's sleep, they have improvement in their self-esteem, their confidence levels go up, and their relationship with their partners and significant others also improve. Let's just say they have a better quality of life when it is more fun down there!

Medications with Sexual Side Effects

Antihypertensives: Alpha-blockers, beta-blockers (e.g., propranolol Δ libido), calcium channel blockers (genital pain or Δ libido), diuretics (spironolactone Δ libido), methyldopa (Δ libido), reserpine (Δ libido), clonidine (Δ libido)
Chemotherapeutic agents: busulfan, cyclophosphamide (Δ arousal, infertility)
Hormonally active agents: Oral contraceptives (Δ libido), antiestrogens/estrogens/selective estrogen receptor modulators, antiandrogens, spironolactone, cimetidine (Δ libido)
Antidepressants: SSRIs (fluoxetine Δorgasm), tricyclic antidepressants (e.g., imiparmine Δ orgasm while clomipramine Δ both libido and orgasm), lithium (Δ libido) MAO-I (isocarboxazid or phenelzine Δ orgasm) Trazadone (painful clitoral tumescence)
Anticholinergic agents, over-the-counter meds, herbals, H2 blockers (e.g., cimetidine (Δ libido), methazolamide for glaucoma (Δ libido)
Antipsychotics: Butyrophenones, phenothiazines (Δ libido)
Carbamazepine, phenytoin, phenobarbital, diazepam (Δ orgasm)
Amphetamines (Δ orgasm)
Narcotics (e.g., methadone, oxycodone Δ orgasm)
Bromocriptine (painful clitoral tumescence)

Δ = "change in" a function; either delayed, decreased, or lack of

Women's Sexual Wellness Quiz

The following questions can help determine if you are having sexual difficulties.

1. Do you become mentally excited during sexual situations (whether alone, stimulating a partner, or being stimulated)?

2. Do you experience genital sensations (tingling, pulsing, swelling) during sexual situations?

3. Do you experience adequate genital lubrication during sexual situations?

4. Do you experience orgasms (alone or with a partner)?

5. Do you experience feelings of guilt after intercourse?

6. Do you feel inferior because of sexual problems?

7. Do you feel that your sexual functioning has negatively affected your personal relationships?

8. Do you suffer incontinence during intercourse?

9. Does your partner suffer from difficulties in sexual functioning?

10. Do you experience pain during intercourse?

Answering *no* to questions 1-4 or *yes* to questions 5-10 may signal a need for intervention.

Take this opportunity to talk to your doctor.

Modified with permission from Dr. Sandep Mistry, Austin, Texas.

Credible Resources on FSD

Goldstein A, Brandon M. *Reclaiming Desire: 4 Keys to Finding Your Lost Libido,* Rodale, 2004

Herbenick D. *Because It Feels Good: A Woman's Guide to Sexual Pleasure and Satisfaction*, Rodale, 2009

Moynihan R, Mintzes B. *Sex, Lies, and Pharmaceuticals: How Drug Companies Plan to Profit from Female Sexual Dysfunction*, Greystone Books, 2010

Berman J, Berman L, Bumiller E. *For Women Only, Revised Edition: A Revolutionary Guide to Reclaiming Your Sex Life,* Henry Holt, 2005

Kaschak E, Tiefer L. *A New View of Women's Sexual Problems*, Haworth Press, 2001

Barbach L. *For Each Other: Sharing Sexual Intimacy*, New York: Signet, 2001

Foley S. *Sex Matters for Women: A Complete Guide to Taking Care of Your Sexual Self,* The Guilford Press, 2002

Winks C, Semans A. *The Good Vibrations Guide to Sex: The Most Complete Sex Manual Ever Written, 3rd Ed,* Cleis Press, 2002

Schnarch D, Maddock J. *Resurrecting Sex: Solving Sexual Problems and Revolutionizing Your Relationship*, Harper Collins, 2003

Zaslau S. *Dx/Rx: Sexual Dysfunction in Men and Women*, Jones and Bartlett, 2011

Some websites that provide support for those who have been sexually abused:

http://www.vawnet.org (National Online Resource Center on Violence Against Women)

http://www.nsvrc.org (National Sexual Violence Resource Center)

http://www.naesv.org (National Alliance to End Sexual Violence Foundation)

http://www.ivatcenters.org (Institute on Violence, Abuse, and Trauma)

http://www.aafp.org/afp/2002/1101/p1705.html (American Family Physician article)

http://www.baylorcme.org/cme/fsd/slides/cme_pdf/talk048.pdf (Diagnosis and Classification of Female Sexual Dysfunction)

Chapter Nine

When Things Stop Working Down There: Menopause and Hormone Replacement Therapy

Didi is a 50-year-old librarian. She believes that ever since she stopped having her period over a year ago, her mood, spirit, and nerves have been out of whack. She has difficulty sleeping, and she has lost her appetite for even foods she used to love. She feels like she is always tired and doesn't have the energy or interest in her hobbies anymore. In fact, her "nerves" are so bad that she can't even concentrate enough to catalogue books at the library. She has stopped seeing her friends. They are concerned because she seems gloomy, and they want her to see a doctor.

Menopause is a normal and natural outcome that eventually happens for all women. Strictly speaking, menopause is when the eggs in a woman's ovaries have become depleted and she stops having periods for one year. In reality, it makes more sense to use the term *perimenopause* to refer to the menopausal transition because the cessation of the period, the waning of the hormones, and the other symptoms do not happen all at once. Hormone levels go up and down and up and down (erratically fluctuating) over a period of several months to years as a woman transitions into menopause.

However, women do continue to make androgens (the male hormones). The average age of menopause is 51.4 years, but there is a range of ages when menopause occurs. Most women will have symptoms during this transition, but there are some fortunate women who may have no symptoms at all. Mary and Georgia are good friends and active members of a local book club. They are both 60 years old, and besides the love of reading mystery novels, they both have many things in common (each has four children and 10 grandchildren, and both love to sail and knit). During one of their many discussions about their changing health, Georgia tells Mary that she can't remember when she went through menopause. The only symptom that is even close to what she has read about (or what she has heard from other friends) is that she had dryness and itching down there, but that went away soon after her doctor gave her estrogen cream. Mary can't believe what she's hearing. For her, menopause turned her life upside down! "Even my joints ache more since menopause," she says.

Carrie is a 44-year-old TV news anchor, who, after years of a regular menstrual cycle with moderate monthly bleeding, now describes having very heavy periods occurring every 20 to 25 days for the past three months. At night she also has started to feel very hot and sweaty near her chest, neck, and face, prompting her to lower the temperature of the air conditioner in her house. She feels tired all the time, and her lack of energy has started to affect her work.

When she asks her doctor what is going on, her doctor asked her when her mother entered menopause. Not surprisingly, Carrie's mother started her menopausal symptoms around the same age and stopped having her periods by age 46. Carrie was surprised but not alarmed to get this news.

Consider another case. Janelle is a 55-year-old mother of three who has been experiencing severe hot flashes and night sweats for five months. She is not able to get a good night's sleep because of these symptoms. She has had pain with intercourse for more than a year. She feels so dry down there that every time she and her husband have sex, it feels like sandpaper inside and burns for hours afterward. She also told us that she seems to get urinary tract infections all the time.

The typical perimenopausal period begins in a woman in her late forties when she starts having irregular menstrual periods. Menstrual periods may come more frequently, less frequently, or may stop for a while and begin again a few months later. Some women even have spotting between their periods. Although, when menopausal, she will stop having periods altogether, the hot flashes and other bothersome symptoms may continue for a number of years after her periods have stopped. After one year of having her last period, she is considered "in menopause."

These natural events can be troubling and disturbing, but there are a number of ways to offset the symptoms so they don't upset your entire life.

In other words, it's very possible to go through menopause gracefully and without creating physical and emotional turmoil in your life.

What Menopause Really Means

Imagine a pregnant woman, more than halfway through her pregnancy, bearing in her belly a little girl, a developing fetus. At this point in pregnancy, the developing female fetus has several million cells within the ovary. Very few of these cells will become eggs during a woman's life. A little girl is born with about 2 million potential eggs, or immature follicles, in her ovaries; but she will only have fewer than 400,000 left by the time she starts puberty. Compare this to at least 20 million sperm that are released by a man *each* time he ejaculates. Huge difference! A woman is born with all the potential eggs she is ever going to have, and she will not be able to make new ones during her lifetime.

During the menstrual cycle, a group of these immature follicles becomes stimulated by hormones, which include follicle-stimulating hormone (FSH) and then luteinizing hormone (LH). Both FSH and LH are released from the pituitary gland, which is located at the base of the woman's brain. The strongest follicle out of the group of stimulated follicles will become a mature egg with the potential of creating a baby if a sperm fertilizes it. All the other one thousand or so neighboring follicles die each month. In fact, approximately 1,000 follicles die during each menstrual cycle until there are zero follicles left, which is the actual reason for menopause. As you can imagine, this process repeats itself each month throughout a woman's reproductive lifetime. As a woman ages, both the quantity as well as the quality of the remaining eggs diminishes. This is why it gets harder for a woman to have children as she becomes older. The stimulated follicles also produce estrogen. Therefore, when the vast majority of the follicles within the ovaries become depleted throughout her lifetime, the estrogen levels also diminish, and this leads to the symptoms of menopause.

Symptoms of Menopause

The symptoms of menopause vary. Some women experience only a few months of hot flashes and night sweats, some experience only a few months of irritability and still others don't experience even a bump in the road. Let's take a look at the most common symptoms and what you can do about them.

Hot Flashes and Night Sweats

Three women with three different experiences of hot flashes are as follows:

- Marla feels heat from the center of the body, radiating outward toward her head and arms, but her feet remain cool. Her forehead and arms get sweaty, and surprisingly, her sinuses open up and clear during hot flashes. She is careful to avoid hot drinks because they will make her have a hot flash.
- Christina says her hot flashes are brought on by either stress or physical activity. She gets dizzy, and her face and neck turn red. The heat from the flashes is so hot that it takes her breath away.
- Victoria doesn't understand what all the fuss is about. She doesn't really experience heat in her sternum or face but does feel her heart beat faster during flashes. And like her Japanese mother, during a hot flash, she feels like her feet are on fire.

Not all women will experience hot flashes, but three out of four will, with one out of 10 experiencing them through their seventies. A hot flash is a sudden feeling of heat in the face and upper chest area, which can spread throughout the body. This occurs because the blood vessels in these areas become dilated and blood flow to these areas increases. Some women may also sweat during hot flashes. In fact, when the hot flashes occur during sleep, they are known as night sweats. These usually occur during the first few hours of sleep, and as you may have guessed, they can make it difficult to get a good night's sleep. Other associated symptoms of menopause include heart palpitations, anxiety, and chills. Hot flashes usually last about three minutes, but in some women, they may last longer. Hot flashes can occur as often as every hour, only a few times per day, once a day, or not at all. Hot flashes typically last for one to two years as your body adjusts to the shift in hormones. However, in some women, they can last for many years.

Why do hot flashes occur? The hypothalamus and insular area of cortex, areas in the brain involved in thermoregulation, are almost addicted to the estrogen that is produced by the ovaries. When the eggs in the ovary are depleted and the estrogen levels decline, these areas of the brain go through withdrawal symptoms, and the results are hot flashes.

Sleep Problems and Depression

In addition to hot flashes and night sweats, some women experience problems falling asleep or staying asleep. Sleep problems may occur even in the absence of night sweats. Waking up few times each night can create havoc the next day. Some women experience irritability, mood changes, nervousness, and trouble concentrating. Others may feel as though they have a permanent case of PMS. In fact, women who have severe PMS in their 30's and 40's tend to have more severe symptoms during perimenopause.

If the emotional roller coaster and sadness become more severe, it can lead to disinterest in normal activities, sadness, and other symptoms of clinical depression. Usually, women who have a history of depression are more prone to experience these severe symptoms during the menopausal transition. Compared to when she was premenopausal, a woman is more than four times as likely to have symptoms of depression during perimenopause and menopause.

Vaginal Dryness, Lack of Libido, Urinary Problems, and Pain with Intercourse

The reduction in hormones that occurs during menopause can have a tremendous impact on your sex life as well as your urinary system. The tissues in the vagina and urethra (the opening where urine exits the bladder) are dependent on estrogen to remain pink, moist, soft, pliable, acidic (a lowered pH), and healthy. However, as hormone levels decline, these sensitive areas become thin, pale, shrunken, and tender to the touch. In fact, the entire length and diameter of the vagina can shrink. The urethra, the tube at the front of vagina that transports urine from the bladder to the outside of the body, also loses its ability to close completely, and the bladder can become more irritable and overactive and may have the symptoms of a urinary tract infection even though there isn't one! When the urethra fails to close completely, urinary incontinence can occur. The areas around the clitoris and the lips can also lose sensation. Intimacy becomes less fulfilling. The declining levels of hormones can affect her desire to have intercourse and make sex uncomfortable and painful (see Chapter Five for further details).

Menopause After a Hysterectomy

How do you know you are going through menopause if you don't have a uterus? Many women have undergone a hysterectomy for a variety of reasons (see Chapter Ten). These women will not experience the typical menstrual symptoms of menopause or changes in their period. However, when the ovaries stop producing estrogen, hot flashes and night sweats may be the first sign of entering the menopausal transition.

Less Common Concerns about Menopause

For women, one of the most concerning changes that can occur as a result of menopause is the loss of the smooth, unwrinkled appearance of their skin. The reduction in estrogen levels throughout the body can lead to loss of the collagen in the skin. Collagen is the connective tissue that provides elasticity and suppleness of the tissues. Additionally, aches and pains throughout the body may increase in both frequency and severity. These include headaches and breast and joint pains. For your doctor, the most concerning changes of menopause include impairment in your sense of balance and bone loss. Together, these changes can put you at higher risk of falling and breaking your hip. A single fall in a patient with osteoporosis can have devastating consequences in a woman's quality of life and may even lead to her early demise.

Although the average age of menopause is 51.4 years, there are some women who are at higher risk for having menopause at a younger age. On average, smokers go through menopause two years earlier than nonsmokers. For reasons not entirely understood, Asian women tend to transition into menopause at an older age than Caucasian women. Those who have a family history (mother, grandmother, and sister) of earlier onset of menopause are likely to go through menopause at a younger age. Finally, women who have never had children tend to have menopause at an earlier age.

Symptoms that Mean Something Else

There are several instances when symptoms like the ones described above are not considered normal. If you are experiencing any of the following, then you should see your doctor immediately:

- Having even a drop of blood from your vagina a year after your period has stopped can be a sign of endometrial cancer, or cancer inside your uterus. Your doctor will need to evaluate this with either an ultrasound or endometrial biopsy.
- Heavy vaginal bleeding during the menopausal transition or any other time in your life may be harmful and lead to anemia and dizziness. Although usually the bleeding is because of hormonal fluctuations, it is always important to rule out cancer or blood diseases as the cause of vaginal bleeding.
- If your periods stop before you are 40 years old, this is called premature ovarian failure. You should see your doctor to get genetic and other testings. On the other hand, if you have infrequent periods before 40, then it is possible that you have a hormone problem such as thyroid disease or polycystic ovarian syndrome (PCOS).
- Certain medication effects can mimic menopausal symptoms such as sweating and flushing. These medications include (Lupron), nicotinic acid, diltiazem, levodopa, alcohol, bromocriptine, amyl nitrite, and excessive thyroid hormone (e.g., Synthroid). Additionally, certain conditions can also mimic some of the symptoms of menopause. These include endocrine problems (including high or low thyroid or high prolactin), adrenal tumor, or cancer.

It is probably not necessary that your doctor perform any blood tests to see if you are going through menopause. If you're in your mid-forties to-fifties and are having the symptoms we described above, then a confirmatory test isn't necessary. During the menopausal transition, blood levels of your hormones do not provide proof that menopause is occurring because the hormones of interest all fluctuate during this period. For example, if you measure hormone levels at some point in time, they may be abnormal. However, if you measure them again one month later, they all may be perfectly normal.

If I'm going through menopause,
do I have to worry about birth control?

Although you are less likely to become pregnant if you are older than mid-forties, it is still possible. You should consider using some form of birth control (either a pill, patch, IUD, diaphragm, or other method) if you're not in menopause. The advantage of hormonal birth control (if you are a candidate) is that it will help regulate your periods also.

What You Can Do

Although we refer to them as symptoms, all things that happen as a woman goes through the menopausal transition are considered a normal part of a woman's life. Menopause is not a disease. In fact, in some cultures (present-day Mayan and Bengali), women don't treat the symptoms of menopause, they embrace it. They just live with the inconveniences and eventually the symptoms go away without any treatment. In the United States, only one in five women with menopausal symptoms seek help from a health professional. On the other hand, if you are experiencing menopausal symptoms and they are making your life difficult or miserable and impacting your quality of life, then you should make an appointment with your gynecologist or primary care doctor.

Before we discuss hormones and medications to treat menopausal symptoms, we would like to mention some ways that you can dampen the uncomfortable feelings of the menopausal transition. First and foremost, educate yourself about menopause. Since you're reading this book, you are already ahead of the game! You can also learn more by visiting the following credible websites: www.menopause.org and www.nlm.nih.gov/medlineplus/menopause.html.

Exercise Regularly

You should try to do moderate exercise for 150 minutes each week. This means 25 minutes six days a week, or you can do 50 minutes three times per week. There are so many benefits of exercise in addition to alleviating the symptoms of menopause. For example, during exercise, your body releases chemicals such as endorphins and growth hormone that can make you feel good and will help fight aging. Exercise can strengthen your cardiovascular system and your bones. Weight-bearing exercises reduce your risk of osteoporosis. Exercise also has been shown to help maintain weight loss and reduce stress, which can help smooth over menopausal mood swings.

Keep Your Bedroom Cool

Something as easy as reducing the temperature in your bedroom can have a tremendous effect on your sleep. Cooler temperature may prevent night sweats. The worse that can happen is that your husband/partner may need to get an extra set of covers!

Avoid Alcohol

Alcohol affects many chemical messengers, or neurotransmitters, in the brain. It can affect your mood, and it may make your depression worse.

Avoid Triggers of Hot Flashes

Emotional stress, hot drinks, and warm areas and humidity may provoke your hot flashes

Relieve Your Stress

Besides exercise, meditation, yoga, creative outlets, and other stress-relief techniques can help you feel better (see Chapter Thirteen for a complete description).

Get Support

Try to stay connected to your friends and family. Friends, especially those who are also going through the same thing, can help you. Emotional support can help you get through menopause gracefully.

Supplements

If you go to a nutrition or health food store and ask them about "natural" alternatives to hormones, they will tout the benefits of vitamin E, evening primrose oil, black cohosh, red clover, flaxseed, soybeans, chickpeas, lentils, and Chinese herbs for treatment of menopausal symptoms. You may even have friends who swear by one or several of these herbal supplements. On the other hand, doctors and scientists are cautious when it comes to these remedies because several studies where unaware (i.e., blinded) subjects were given either a placebo, sugar pill, or the natural remedy did not show that these relieve menopause symptoms. We are not convinced of their benefits either. Table 1 lists some of the natural and alternative remedies that have been studied and also the strength of scientific evidence behind their use.

Table 1. **Alternatives Remedies for Down There Conditions**

Supplement	Derived from	Potential Adverse/Toxic Effects	Conditions Treated (as advertised)	Is It Effective Based on Scientific Evidence?
Ginseng	Plant, *Panax ginseng*	None	Low sexual desire	NB
			Immunity	???
			Weight loss	NB
			Hot flashes	NB
			Stress	???
			Fatigue	???
			Cancer fighting	???
Soy and plant estrogens	Miso, tofu, soy, flaxseed, red clover	May stimulate breast tissue in breast cancer patients	Vaginal dryness, causing pain during intercourse	?B
			Hot flashes	B*
			High cholesterol	?B*
Black cohosh	Plant, *Actaea racemosa*	May be confused with blue cohosh, which can be toxic	Hot flashes	?B
			Sleep problems	???
			Anxiety and depression	???
			Painful menstruation	???
			PMS	???
St. John's wort	flower, *Hypericum perforatum*	Side effects of constipation and dry mouth, may increase cataract risk, interacts with other medications, may amplify sun's effect on skin	Mild depression	B
			Severe depression	???

Evening primrose	Flower oil	None	Painful breasts	???
			PMS	NB
			Hot flashes	NB
			Urinary urgency and bladder problems	???
Dong quai	*Angelica sinensis* root	Blood thinner, may interact with other medications, may amplify sun's effect on skin	Hot flashes	NB
			Regulating menstrual cycles	???
			High blood pressure	???
			Fatigue	???
Valerian	Plant root	May cause rapid heartbeat, heart failure, confusion	Sleep aid	NB
			Sedative	NB
Wild yam	Plant vine containing *Dioscorea*	Paradoxically, "Mexican yam" may have estrogen properties, thus caution in breast cancer patients	Menstrual cramps	NB
			Hot flashes	NB
			Gallbladder problems	???
Chasteberry	Plant, *Vitex agnus-castus*		Low sexual desire	???
			Breast pain	???
			PMS	???
			Depression	???
			Vaginal dryness	???

NB = no benefit
??? = we don't know yet
? B = possibly beneficial (weak evidence)
B = definitely beneficial (strong evidence)
* = beneficial in sufficient quantities

Hormone Replacement Therapy

Studies of estrogen have demonstrated a beneficial effect for relief of menopausal symptoms. Nonestrogen treatments, especially antidepressant medications, also have been shown to be effective for the treatment of menopausal symptoms. However, nothing is as effective as the real thing, estrogen. (see Table 2).

Table 2. **The Scientific Evidence for Impact of Estrogen and Other Medicines for the Treatment of Menopausal Symptoms**

Type of Remedy/Treatment	Beneficial	Neutral (no harm/no benefit)	Harmful
Estrogen	yes		*
Progestin	yes		
Clonidine	yes		
Gabapentin (Neurontin)	yes		
Paroxetine (Paxil)	yes		
Sertraline (Zoloft)		yes	
Fluoxetine (Prozac)	yes		
Venlafaxine (Effexor)	yes		

* = breast cancer stimulation risk

Simply put, oral estrogen, plus progestin, has been linked to higher risks of blood clots. This became evident after the results of a large, influential studies, named the Women's Health Initiative (WHI), were published. Unfortunately, the media and some who didn't understand how to interpret the study results exaggerated the negative findings and omitted the positive ones. Overall, a negative spin was put in the headlines, and hormone replacement therapy (HRT) was demonized.

With that in mind, we have provided you with an objective overview of the WHI study so that you can understand it and make up your own mind about whether you want to use hormones or not. The WHI was a series of scientific studies, two of which were designed to determine the effects of hormones on women's hearts. The initial results were published in 2002. In the first study, about 16,000 women who had a uterus (i.e., had not had a hysterectomy) were randomly assigned to taking daily estrogen plus progestin or placebo. The women who chose to participate in this study did not know whether the pill they were taking contained active hormones or was a harmless sugar pill. Thus, they were blinded to which pill they were taking. In the second study, about 11,000 women who had already had a hysterectomy were assigned to either estrogen only or placebo. Both of these studies were stopped earlier than their intended duration because of an increased rate of adverse events. The bullets below simplify and summarize the results of the WHI studies. We have listed the main points:

- In the first WHI study, comparing conjugated equine estrogen (E) plus medroxyprogesterone acetate (P), or E+P, to sugar pill (placebo), there was both a risk as well as benefit incurred by using hormones E+P.
- Patients who took E+P had a higher absolute risk of developing blood clots, strokes, and breast cancers. However, the increased risk of stroke and breast cancer was small. There may be a slightly higher risk of new or early breast cancer but the risk of dying from breast cancer was unchanged.
- Patients who took E+P had a lower risk of developing colon cancer and also had protection from osteoporotic fractures. However, the colon cancer risk reduction was small. There may be a slight reduction in risk of colon cancer.
- When all the statistical analyses were done, the definite conclusion that can be drawn from the first WHI study is that E+P increases the risk of blood clots but reduces the risk of fractures.
- In the second WHI study, comparing just conjugated equine estrogen (E) to a sugar pill (placebo), there was both a risk as well as benefit incurred by using estrogen alone.
- Patients who took estrogen alone had a minimally higher risk of developing strokes.
- Patients who took estrogen alone had lower risk of osteoporotic fractures of the hip and spine.

- When all the statistical analyses of the second WHI study were completed, the definite conclusion that can be drawn is that estrogen, by itself, protects from developing fractures.

The great thing about scientific studies is that if they are well planned, designed, and conducted, then you can have a high degree of confidence in their results. Statisticians are employed to check the calculations to see whether the results are statistically significant. In other words, the statisticians make sure that results did not occur by chance. Another way of saying this is that based on the WHI study, we can be 95 percent confident that estrogen protects against fractures.

The women who took estrogen plus progestin had a higher rate of blood clot; however, they had an even higher rate of protection from fractures. Blood clots in the lung are called pulmonary emboli (PE), and those in the leg are referred to as deep vein thrombosis (DVT). Both of these are dangerous, especially PE. On the other hand, fractures that result from osteoporosis, especially those of the hip, can be devastating to a person's life. "The troubling increase in the death rate in hip fracture patients—from 24 percent in the 1980s to 29 percent in the new Globe study—demands an aggressive response," some researchers said. Hip fractures far too often start a cascade of complications that ends in death. A staggering death toll, but one that receives limited attention.

Fortunately, there are a group of medications called bisphosphonates, which are effective for prevention as well as treatment of osteoporosis. We do not recommend only taking estrogen for the prevention or treatment of osteoporosis and fractures.

Statistically speaking, the increased risks of breast cancer and stroke are weak. When the results are broken down by age, older postmenopausal women (age > 59) did have a higher rate of coronary heart disease and new, early breast cancer. It is important to mention that the risk of both breast cancer and heart disease increases with age even if you don't take hormones. The first WHI study (comparing E+P to placebo), the two things that we can be certain of is that estrogen plus progestin did increase the risk of blood clots, but it also provided substantial benefit by preventing fractures. From the second WHI study (comparing E only to placebo) the one result that we can count on is that estrogen did reduce the risk of bone fractures.

In addition to the above studies, we have learned a lot from other studies that were completed before WHI. These studies indicate that progestin is not all bad and in certain circumstances is necessary. In women who have not had a hysterectomy, estrogen given without progestin can lead to a higher risk of endometrial cancer (or cancer of the lining of the uterus).

In a nutshell:

- You should rely on the big numbers to guide your decisions. The increased blood clot risk and the protection from bone fracture are both true findings that you can hang your hat on.
- Some of the results of the WHI studies cannot be relied on because they occurred by chance (e.g. heart disease risk).
- If you have a uterus and are taking estrogen, you must also take progesterone.
- More scientific studies are needed using estrogen in slightly younger women (i.e. those going through perimenopause) with the primary goal of studying the effects of estrogen on breast cancer in order for us to know whether estrogen actually does increase breast cancer risk in those for whom it is prescribed when needed.

Bioidentical Hormones

Bioidentical hormones are hormones that more closely mimic naturally circulating hormones in a woman's body. Bioidentical hormones are available by prescription from drugstores or they can be specially made by a compounding pharmacist who can take a physician's prescription for a very specific medication, which is unique for a patient's individual needs. Tables 5 and 6 list several examples.

Table 5. **Which Estrogens Are Bioidentical?**

What Is The Brand Name?	Where Is It Derived From?	Type Of Estrogen (chemical substance)	Is This Considered Bioidentical?	Does It Come in Pill, Cream, Gel, or Patch Form?
Estrace	Plants	17β estradiol	Yes	Pill, vaginal cream
Climara and Vivelle	Plants	17β estradiol	Yes	Patch

EstroGel	Plants	17β estradiol	Yes	Gel
Cenestin and Enjuvia	Plants	Synthetic conjugated estrogens	No	Pill
Premarin (used in WHI)	Urine of pregnant mare (horse)	Conjugated equine estrogens	No	Pill
Any birth control pill	Synthetic	Ethinyl estradiol	No	Pill

Table 6. **Which Progestogens Are Bioidentical?**

What Is The Brand Name?	What Is It Derived From?	Type Of Progestogen	Is This Considered Bioidentical?	Does It Come In A Gel Or Pill?
Prometrium	Plants	Micronized progesterone	Yes	Pill
Prochieve and Crinone	Plants	Micronized progesterone	Yes	Vaginal gel
Provera (used in WHI)	Synthetic	Medroxyprogesterone acetate	No	Pill
Micronor, Loestrin, and other birth control pills	Synthetic	Norethindrone	No	Pill
Ovral and other birth control pills	Synthetic	Norgestrel	No	Pill

Bioidentical hormones have been touted by celebrities who have claimed that the hormones have antiaging properties, counteract stress, increase metabolism, increase good cholesterol, and decrease the risk of breast cancer. There are no drugs, compounds, or elixirs that are this perfect. These bioidentical hormones have not yet been scientifically proven to correct all these conditions. Many of these preparations have not been well studied, and thus, they are likely to have the same risks and benefits as non-bioidentical hormones. The two tables above give examples of FDA-approved and regulated bioidentical hormones. If you choose to go to a compounding pharmacist to get that perfect mixture of estradiol and progestin for your body, realize that compounded preparations are not regulated or FDA-approved, the dosing can be inconsistent from batch to batch, and safety has not been studied. Also, there is no proof that compounded hormones are more effective in relieving menopausal symptoms than the bioidentical hormones listed above.

On the other hand, compounding may be useful when your doctor wants to prescribe a mixture of several hormones, certain doses of hormones that are unique for each woman, or a type of hormone (for example, testosterone) that is not readily available. Doctors who are comfortable with using compounded hormones will often perform a blood test to check levels of various hormones and substances in your bloodstream. They can then prescribe the precise dose of cream or elixir in order to replace the deficient hormone and return the blood levels to the normal range.

Our Recommendations

As you can tell by reading the tables that we have provided in this chapter, it can be difficult to understand exactly how estrogen and progestin affect womens' bodies. The studies can be difficult to interpret, even for doctors. And given that the media is often interested in sensationalizing a story, it is no wonder that the facts from the WHI study were not presented in an objective manner. Unfortunately, much of the media interpretation of the WHI studies has been inaccurate and misleading, creating a lot of unnecessary fear and panic among millions of women. Millions of women stopped using hormones overnight. We base our counseling of patients regarding estrogen and hormone therapy not only on the results of the WHI study, but on findings of other studies as well. We individualize our recommendations. A discussion with your doctor about your risks of heart disease, blood clots, breast cancer, and bone fractures is necessary before making the decision to use or not use hormone therapy. This is the purpose of this book: to provide you with the important information and allow you and your doctor to make an informed decision regarding the use of hormone replacement therapy.

For us, the WHI doesn't address a few areas. Did the higher rate of blood clots, the questionably higher rate of breast cancer, and the increased risk of stroke occur because of the type of hormone or the dose used in the study, or because the study participants were much older than the typical patients for whom most gynecologists prescribe hormones? Maybe it was a combination of all these elements. The type of estrogen given to the study participants was conjugated equine estrogen (which is derived from a pregnant mare or horse estrogen). The type of progestin used in the WHI was medroxyprogesterone acetate (a synthetic progestin). The dose of hormones used in the WHI was 0.625 mg of estrogen and 2.5 mg of progestin. These hormones were taken orally, which results in a different type of metabolism within the body and, as a result, increases the likelihood of blood thickening—thus potential for blood clots or DVT and PE. Some studies suggest that the transdermal application of these hormones is safer than oral preparations when it comes to cardiovascular and clotting risk. The transdermal may have fewer adverse effects because the drug goes from the skin directly into the bloodstream, whereas the medication taken orally has to pass from the gastrointestinal tract to the liver where it is metabolized. This processing stimulates proteins (such as clotting factors and activated protein C) associated with stroke and heart disease.

In a nutshell, here's an overview of the main takeaways regarding hormone therapy and menopause:

- The WHI studies did not answer several questions.
- Does estrogen +/- progestin have the same effects in younger patients such as those women in their late forties and early fifties, who are just starting to go through menopause?
- Is there a difference between oral estrogen (used in WHI) and other forms of estrogen (e.g., cream, patch, or spray)?
- Is there a difference between bioidentical hormones and the type of hormones used in WHI?
- Our recommendations are the following: The use of low-dose transdermal bioidentical estrogen is safe and useful in women in their forties and fifties who are suffering from menopausal symptoms that affect their quality of life. If you are over 60, you still may be a candidate for estrogen. You should discuss this option with your doctor.

If a patient has moderate to severe menopausal symptoms, we prescribe the lowest dose of estrogen that helps relieve her symptoms. We consider symptoms of high-enough severity to warrant treatment when they interfere with your quality of life. Some women may have severe hot flashes but may cope and just live with them. On the other hand, others may have a hot flash once a week, but it is so bothersome that they seek treatment. Only you know how bad things feel inside and whether you are a candidate for treatment. But you must convey to your physician the impact of these symptoms on your quality of life. Only then can your doctor help to restore you to a level of normalcy.

For women who have moderate to severe hot flashes and diminished quality of life, we will often prescribe a transdermal method of absorbing estrogen instead of an oral tablet. This can be accomplished with a patch, cream, or spray. You may choose the method that suits you best. For instance, many patients seem to like the patch because they only have to change it twice per week. In that instance, we would prescribe a low-dose (0.025 mg/day or 0.0375 mg/day) estradiol patch, which is plant derived, FDA approved, and a consistent formulation that is readily available. If low dose doesn't relieve your symptoms, then your doctor can increase the dose. We recommend using it for a short period of time (less than five years) to resolve symptoms. For those who have not had a hysterectomy, we will give low-dose transdermal estrogen and insert a progestin-containing intrauterine device (Mirena IUD) to protect the endometrium. For patients who don't want an IUD, we may give a micronized progesterone tablet or cream. Additionally, we feel more comfortable and confident in prescribing these hormones for women who are within 10 years of menopause (about less than 60 years old). If you're older than 60, then you should discuss the risks and benefits of hormone therapy with your doctor, as you are still a candidate. We would also recommend routine mammograms and breast self-exams for anyone using this regimen.

It may be useful for you to know that the following estrogens have similar potency:

0.625 mg conjugated equine estrogens $\approx$
50 mcg/day (0.050 mg/day) transdermal 17β estradiol $\approx$
1 mg micronized 17β estradiol $\approx$
1.25 mg Piperazine estrone sulfate $\approx$
1/6th birth control pill containing 30 mcg ethinyl estradiol

What You Can Expect from Hormone Therapy

After taking hormones for a few days, you should notice improvement in some of the menopausal symptoms described above. Younger menopausal women with bothersome symptoms can expect to have reduction in hot flashes and may notice improvement in sleep, mood, and depression. Some studies have shown an improvement in balance and stability as well as improvement in skin texture and tone. But keep in mind that no two women will have the same response from therapy. Although many women (those who haven't had a hysterectomy) who take estrogen plus progestin therapy will have irregular spotting or bleeding during the first few months of therapy, by six months, most women will completely stop having periods. Some women also experience breast tenderness. For those whose bleeding does not respond to adjustment in the dose of one of the hormones (usually progestin), they should return to their doctor for evaluation and dosage adjustment of the medication. If you are postmenopausal and have irregular bleeding, your doctor will probably want to rule out endometrial cancer by doing a transvaginal ultrasound or an endometrial biopsy. The transvaginal ultrasound is performed by placing a thin ultrasound probe inside the vagina and scanning the uterus to ensure that the endometrium (inner lining of the uterus) is not too thick. If, however, the ultrasound is not diagnostic to exclude cancer, then your doctor will want to obtain a biopsy of the endometrium. This can be done in the office and takes less than a minute, but the procedure itself can cause some cramping.

Medical Options without HRT

For those who do not want or cannot take hormones for menopausal symptoms, they should consider Neurontin, Paxil, Prozac, Effexor, Pristiq, or clonidine. It is not recommended that a patient with a history of an estrogen receptor-positive breast cancer take any form of estrogen because it may stimulate cancer cells. Neurontin is approved for treatment of seizures but has been used for other purposes, such as pain and hot flashes. Paxil, Effexor, Prozac, and Pristiq are all unique antidepressant medications (but not all antidepressants are effective for hot flashes). For example, Zoloft is in the same medication family as Paxil and Prozac and yet is not effective for menopausal symptoms. Neurontin, Effexor, or Paxil is our choice of nonhormonal treatment of hot flashes, but these medications need to be taken for at least one month before significant improvement occurs. Clonidine also is effective but the side effects, consisting of low blood pressure and dizziness, decreased sex drive, and drowsiness, may hamper its value.

Patients Who Should Not Take Estrogen

Patients who have breast cancer, a history of blood clots, stroke, active liver disease, or coronary heart disease, or who are at high risk (such as lupus, active gallbladder disease, and blood disorder that makes your blood too thick) for having any of these medical conditions should not take estrogens. In addition, if you are older than 35 years and are having irregular periods, we would not recommend that you take birth control pills if you are a smoker. A typical birth control pill has at least six times the potency of estrogen than the amount of estrogen in HRT for menopausal symptoms. The risk of blood clotting goes up in these women, and the benefits do not outweigh the risks.

Considerations When Taking HRT

There are a few conditions that may be adversely affected by oral estrogen and progestin, and for which we do not recommend taking HRT.

- Gallbladder disease—harmful, hormone may increase risk of cholecystitis (inflammation of gallbladder) and need for gallbladder removal
- Urinary incontinence—harmful; worsens incontinence; however, local or vaginal estrogen provided with a topical vaginal cream or a suppository may be beneficial
- Diabetes mellitus (type 2)—beneficial, hormone may reduce your body's resistance to insulin
- Asthma—don't know, conflicting evidence
- Epilepsy—don't know, not enough evidence
- Systemic lupus erythematosus—harmful, may increase risk of flare in women with lupus
- Migraine—don't know, conflicting evidence

- Overall mortality—beneficial, hormones may reduce mortality (especially in women younger than 60). Additionally, women younger than 60 who retain their ovaries at the time of hysterectomy have lower mortality. For women under age 65, who are not at high risk for ovarian or breast cancer and who are having a hysterectomy for benign reasons, we recommend preservation of both ovaries (see Chapter Ten).

The Bottom Line

Menopause and HRT are not straightforward. Hormones have a multitude of effects on your body. Menopausal women should have a frank discussion with their doctor regarding their symptoms. They should also discuss their concerns and needs. If menopause is affecting your quality of life, then postmenopausal hormone therapy may be appropriate for you as long as you don't have contraindications. Don't wait. Talk to your doctor now.

Chapter Ten

When a Hysterectomy
Is the Right Choice . . . or Not

More than a half million hysterectomies are performed every year in the United States, which is far fewer than just a few years ago. Why the decline? More alternatives to hysterectomy are now available, and more women are educated about these options. Because of our amazing and constant access to information on the Web, informed women are choosing to forego having a hysterectomy when there isn't a good reason for having the procedure. Women are also more inclined to ask for a second opinion when they do not agree with their doctor's recommendation or are not comfortable with it.

Oftentimes a hysterectomy is not necessary, but sometimes, removal of the uterus can be highly beneficial to a woman's quality of life. Consider Carolyn, a 44-year-old mother, who has had two children by vaginal deliveries. She has had excessive vaginal bleeding and very painful menstrual periods for many years. She has a family history of breast cancer and has had a breast biopsy for a suspicious lesion noted on a mammogram a month ago. Her gynecologist recommended a total hysterectomy, including the removal of her ovaries, which frightened Carolyn. She had a number of questions that she felt were not answered adequately, such as the following: Is there an alternative to hysterectomy? Why do my ovaries need to be removed? Won't I go into menopause if you remove my ovaries? What is the safest, fastest, and least-invasive way to remove my uterus if I have to have it removed? If I have to have a hysterectomy, can I have a partial hysterectomy instead?

When Carolyn spoke to her mom (who had a hysterectomy when she was in her midtwenties), she was advised not to have a hysterectomy "because after I had my hysterectomy, I had the worst hot flashes you can imagine. My hormones went out of whack for years, and your father and I were never intimate like we used to be," her mother said.

Understandably, Carolyn felt anxious as she tried to weigh the pros and cons of going through with this irreversible surgery. As a result, she sought us out for a second opinion.

Even though a hysterectomy is one of the most common operations done on women, with more than one out of every three woman in the United States having a hysterectomy by age 65, deciding on whether or not to go through with this surgery can be very anxiety producing. Many women base their femininity on the presence of an intact uterus, and the removal of a uterus may be psychologically disturbing. Carolyn thought, "I just can't imagine having my reproductive organs removed. I am a woman, and I was born with a uterus and ovaries for a reason. It doesn't seem right to have them removed." But in a woman who is done with childbearing and who has problems caused by her uterus that reduce her quality of life, the removal of a uterus, a hysterectomy, can be of paramount importance to a woman's overall health.

Is Hysterectomy Right for You?

There are six major reasons that determine whether a woman is a candidate for hysterectomy:

1. Cancer or precancerous disease of the reproductive tract is the most straightforward. If you have cancer, then you need to remove all the involved organs and possibly adjacent areas.

2. Pelvic pain is the most confusing and challenging. As you can tell from reading Chapter Five, there are numerous reasons for pelvic pain, and there are no guarantees that removal of the reproductive organs will improve your pelvic pain.

3. Pelvic infection usually occurs from sexually transmitted infections such as gonorrhea and chlamydia; and if recognized at an early stage, then antibiotics are all that is necessary to cure the infection. However, if the

infection progresses to an advanced state, then a hysterectomy may be the only option.

4. Some women have severe uterine bleeding that does not respond to alternative measures such as hormones, D&C, or endometrial ablation. (Endometrial ablation is same thing as destruction by hyperthermia. It is a general term that can include other modalities of destroying the endometrium.)

5. Some women have symptomatic fibroids (e.g., very large uterus causing pressure on your other organs) that do not respond to other measures such as hormones, uterine artery embolization, or myomectomy, or they do not like the other options.

6. It can be an option for women with advanced uterine prolapse (e.g., uterus and other pelvic organs are protruding five inches outside the vagina) who don't want to use a pessary (see Chapter Three for more detail).

Bleeding, fibroids, and prolapse are the most common indications for hysterectomy in the United States. When it comes to managing these three conditions, your doctor first will offer a conservative approach (i.e. , noninvasive) to treat your symptoms. However, if your problem is severe or not responding to other therapies, then a hysterectomy becomes the best option.

When we are counseling our patients regarding all the options available to treat them, hysterectomy is usually not the first choice that we offer a woman. In fact, apart from cases of cancer, only a few hysterectomies are absolutely necessary to save a woman's life. Most hysterectomies are done to improve quality of life, such as to reduce discomfort, pain, or bleeding. Besides, aggressive cancers of the reproductive tract, such as cervical, uterine, and ovarian cancer, the other conditions that can make a hysterectomy absolutely necessary to save a woman's life are uncontrollable bleeding from the vagina and severe pelvic infection.

Prolapse, vaginal bleeding, pelvic pain, and abnormal growths are the most common benign, noncancerous problems that reduce a woman's quality of life. Your doctor may recommend a hysterectomy for these conditions. However, before considering surgical removal of the uterus, there are other nonsurgical solutions that should be tried. As described in Chapter Three, prolapse can be managed conservatively with a pessary. Pelvic pain, if it is caused by endometriosis (where the lining of the uterus grows outside the uterus), can also be managed with hormonal therapy (such as leuprolide hormone [Lupron]). This is described in detail in Chapter Five.

Understanding the Surgery . . . When It Is Necessary

Hysterectomy is a major surgery where the uterus is separated from its blood supply and attachments to the pelvis, separated from the bladder and the rectum, and removed from the body. The removed uterus is dropped into a surgical pan and goes to the lab where a pathologist slices and dices the tissue and looks at it under the microscope to make an accurate diagnosis and to be certain that there is no cancer in the uterus or other condition responsible for your symptoms. The blood vessels to the uterus supply oxygen and nutrients and also carry away waste products. The ligaments, which are like ropes, hold the uterus in place and suspend it in the middle of the pelvis. The ropes wrap around the cervix and hold the sides of the uterus. These all have to be disconnected from your uterus.

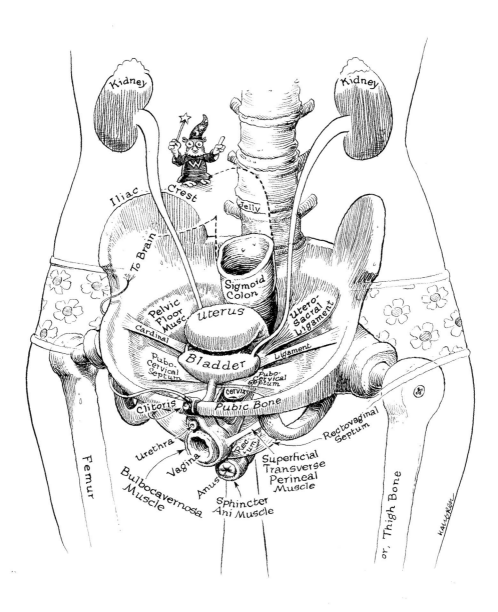

During the operation, all these structures that support and hold the uterus are divided, and the tissue left behind is ligated, or tied off, with strong absorbable suture material. Another crucial step in the operation involves disconnecting the cervix from the vagina. If the hysterectomy is done properly, the vagina is not removed with the cervix and uterus. However, when too much vagina is removed, the length of the vagina can become shorter, and this may result in painful intercourse after the surgery. Although this is an uncommon occurrence, it can be a devastating complication of hysterectomy, especially in the sexually active woman. Painful intercourse is hardly a trade-off for the relief of the symptoms of a fibroid or vaginal bleeding.

Possible Complications of a Hysterectomy

Like any other major surgery, there is a risk of injury to structures surrounding the operative site. During separation of the uterus from the bladder or rectum, an inadvertent cut or injury may be made in these organs. Other organs near the site of surgery such as the bowel and the ureter (tubes leading from the kidney to the bladder) also can be damaged during a hysterectomy. Injury to any of these structures is uncommon, and if it occurs and the injury is recognized, it can be repaired during the procedure with minimal or no consequences after the procedure. However, if injuries to the ureter, bowel, or bladder occur and are not recognized at the time of the hysterectomy, there can be significant complications and even additional surgery. If the blood vessels to the uterus are not adequately sealed, then postoperative bleeding may ensue. If this bleeding is significant, the woman may need a blood transfusion and/or a trip back to the operating room to control the bleeding. Fortunately, very few women will require a blood transfusion after a hysterectomy. However, if a transfusion is required, blood used in the United States is extremely safe. Acquiring an infection is also a possibility after any type of procedure or surgery, and hysterectomy is no exception. Although infection is uncommon after a hysterectomy, the most common areas are inside the bladder or the vagina, which can usually be managed with antibiotics and only delays the recovery period for a few days.

There are also risks associated with having general anesthesia, when a patient is completely asleep. The blood may clot in the leg because of lack of movement of the legs during general anesthesia or after surgery. This is called deep vein thrombosis, or DVT. Sometimes the clot may dislodge from the leg and travel to the lungs, causing a severe, life-threatening problem. This blood clot in the lungs is called pulmonary embolism, or PE. The risks of DVT and PE are extremely low, and your surgeon takes every precaution to reduce the likelihood of these events occurring. For example, a leg massager that regularly squeezes the calves is commonly placed on all patients during and after surgery to prevent blood clots in the leg. Additionally, some patients are given a blood thinner called heparin to reduce the risk of blood clotting.

Finally, although the exact reasons are not currently understood, women who undergo hysterectomy and whose ovaries are not removed may go through menopause a few years earlier than the average age. For example, the average age of menopause in white women is 51. In other words, the ovaries naturally stop making estrogen by age 51; and as a result, a woman may experience menopausal symptoms such as hot flashes, night sweats, etc., as described in Chapter Nine. A white woman who has had a hysterectomy without removal of ovaries may go into menopause at age 49 (about two years earlier). One possibility for this is that the surgery may reduce the blood supply to the ovaries—even though the ovaries themselves are not removed.

Types and Routes of Hysterectomy

- Although the goal is the same—removal of the uterus—there are several ways in which the uterus can be removed.
- All of the procedures and surgeries discussed in this book are described in greater detail in the Glossary of *Down There* Operations, at the end of the book.
- If the entire operation is performed through a five-inch cut near the hairline above the pubic bone (bikini cut), then it is called a total abdominal hysterectomy (TAH). This is the most invasive of all methods (see illustration below).
- If the entire operation is performed through several tiny keyhole incisions in the belly, and the uterus is diced up into tiny pieces and removed through the keyholes, then it is called a total laparoscopic hysterectomy (TLH). If a TLH is performed with the assistance of a surgical robot, it is called a robotic-assisted laparoscopic hysterectomy.
- If a small opening is made inside the vagina and the entire operation is performed through the vagina and no incisions are made in the belly, it is called a transvaginal hysterectomy (TVH). This is the least invasive of all methods. Of all the methods discussed so far and if indicated, it is better for you if your surgeon can perform a vaginal hysterectomy. This type of hysterectomy has the lowest complication rates, the least time under anesthesia, and the fastest recovery rate of all the methods. Even when comparing all the minimally invasive options with each other (see Glossary of *Down There* Operations), TVH is still the winner because it is the safest, it has the shortest operating time, and you can still look great in a bathing suit as the vaginal hysterectomy leaves no unsightly scars on the belly.

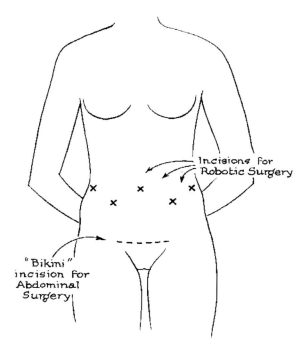

Alternatives to Hysterectomy

There are many circumstances when a hysterectomy is not necessary. Alternatives to hysterectomy are discussed in detail below and also described in the Glossary of *Down There* Operations at the end of the book.

Dilatation and currettage (D&C)

For very heavy and irregular periods, the entire uterine lining may need to be removed or shaved. This procedure is called a hysteroscopy and dilatation and curettage, or D&C. This procedure is done in the operating room while the patient is asleep. The advantage of the D&C or the shaving of the lining of the uterus is that it gives a woman the chance to keep her reproductive organs, is less invasive, and has a shorter recovery time than a total hysterectomy where the whole uterus is removed.

Uterine artery embolization (UAE)

A high-tech treatment option for fibroids, which is done under local anesthesia, is called uterine artery embolization. This procedure can be performed if fibroids are causing abnormal vaginal bleeding or pressure because of their large size and the patient does not want to have surgery.

Small particles are injected into the uterine arteries to block them and thus cut off the blood supply to the offending fibroids. By cutting off the blood supply to the uterus, the fibroids shrink and wither away and many patients have improvement in their symptoms. The biggest disadvantage of this procedure is that a uterine specimen is not obtained, and thus, there is no way to rule out cancer if it exists. After the procedure, pain and cramping are common, and pain medications will be necessary for a period of time, usually less than a week. Some patients may also experience nausea, vomiting, vaginal discharge, weakness, and even fever after the procedure. Although this can be done on an outpatient basis, we recommend an overnight stay in the hospital for management of pain and nausea after the procedure. Also, it is a good idea to stay around town for at least a month after this procedure so you're able to see your doctor if any issues, such as pain or heavy discharge, arise. We do not recommend this procedure in women who wish to have more children as there is not enough scientific evidence for us to recommend that it is safe to have children after having a uterine artery embolization.

Myomectomy

Another treatment option for a fibroid, which allows a woman to keep her uterus, is called a myomectomy. This is a major surgery where one or more fibroids are surgically removed from the uterus. If indicated and done well, most women's symptoms will be resolved. Myomectomy is often chosen either by women who want relief from problems caused by fibroids and want to keep their uterus or those who want to improve their ability to carry a pregnancy, especially if they have had repetitive miscarriages because of fibroids. The downside to myomectomy is that not all fibroids can be removed—small fibroids may remain. These remaining small fibroids or new ones can grow again over time. Additionally, if during the myomectomy, removal of the fibroids requires opening the uterine cavity, then if you become pregnant in the future, a cesarean delivery will be necessary for subsequent childbirth because the uterus now may be too weak to go through labor and a vaginal delivery. It is a good idea to find a surgeon who is skilled in minimally invasive methods of doing a myomectomy (such as laparoscopic, robotic, or in some cases vaginal) because these methods reduce the likelihood of having unwanted adhesions in the abdomen. Adhesions can impair your ability to become pregnant, and in some people, they may be a source of postoperative pain.

Endometrial ablation

If medications fail to help with vaginal bleeding that is a result of hormonal imbalance, then endometrial ablation is an option. This procedure, which often can be done in the doctor's office under local anaesthesia and oral pain medication, is successful in reducing the amount of bleeding and in some it can stop bleeding completely. During endometrial ablation, the lining of the uterus, the endometrium, is heated to a high temperature resulting in its destruction. The procedure is much less invasive than a hysterectomy, is less expensive, and has shorter recovery period. However, the disadvantage is it may not always completely solve the problem of vaginal bleeding. Up to approximately 50 percent of patients who have had this procedure end up requiring another procedure within 10 years, usually a hysterectomy.

Levonorgestrel IUD (Mirena™)

The progestin intrauterine device (Pg-IUD) is the least invasive of all the alternatives to hysterectomy mentioned so far. The Pg-IUD is a small (one inch), T-shaped piece of soft plastic containing the hormone levonorgestrel that can be inserted into the womb during an office procedure without sedation. The Mirena IUD is an effective birth control device that is effective for up to five years. The hormone causes the lining of the uterus to become very thin and thus not bleed. After insertion of the Pg-IUD, your periods will diminish but you may have irregular spotting for the first few months. Some women completely stop having periods. Uncommon side effects of the Pg-IUD are due to the progestin and include headache, breast tenderness, and nausea. Although Mirena was designed as a reversible long-term birth control method, it has been shown to be effective in treatment of heavy menstrual bleeding and menstrual cramps. Studies indicate that the satisfaction rate between Mirena and UAE is similar.

To Remove the Ovaries . . . or Not: Important Considerations

Regardless of the route by which the hysterectomy is performed, removal of the ovaries and Fallopian tubes is not considered part of a hysterectomy. The removal of the ovaries and Fallopian tubes, or bilateral salpingo-oophorectomy, is a separate and distinct procedure from a hysterectomy. However, there are situations, such as cancer of the reproductive tract or severe endometriosis, where both procedures, the hysterectomy and the removal of the ovaries and fallopian tubes, are performed at the same time. In other words, just because you are having a hysterectomy doesn't mean your ovaries have to be removed too. There is usually a broad discrepancy between the patient's description of her hysterectomy and what actually happened during that surgery. When questioned about their surgical histories, most of our patients incorrectly say that they've had a partial hysterectomy when in fact they have had a total hysterectomy—their entire uterus and cervix were removed, but the ovaries were not. When doctors communicate with each other about partial hysterectomy, they mean the uterus is removed, but the cervix and both ovaries were not removed.

The current medical advice is that in a woman who is undergoing hysterectomy for most benign disease, it is beneficial to leave the ovaries and not remove them. Based on recent studies evaluating the risks and benefits, after age 65, there is less need to leave the ovaries in place, and thus removal of the ovaries is not a problem. Premature removal of the ovaries is associated with death at a younger age and higher risk of osteoporosis (see Chapter Nine for more details). However, there are certain circumstances when a woman younger than 65 could consider removing her normal ovaries. If your family has a strong history of ovarian or breast cancer, then the risk of developing ovarian cancer is higher than that of the average person. Additionally, if a woman is having a hysterectomy (for one of the aforementioned reasons) but also has severe premenstrual syndrome (PMS), endometriosis, epilepsy, or migraine headaches that are triggered by monthly menstrual cycles, then she may consider removing both ovaries at the time of hysterectomy regardless of age. Young women who have not yet undergone menopause (premenopausal women) who have had both of their ovaries removed at the time of hysterectomy should take estrogen as it is definitely safe to take in this circumstance.

Hysterectomy or Partial Hysterectomy: Which Should You Have?

The word *total* in TAH or TLH means the entire uterus is removed including the cervix. Sometimes either the patient or the doctor prefers to remove the uterus but leave behind the cervix. This procedure is called a supracervical hysterectomy (SCH), which is truly a partial hysterectomy. Several decades ago, it was the opinion of the medical community that the removal of the cervix may lead to disruption of the sensory nerves and the support structure of the vagina. SCH may take less time to perform, but it has disadvantages. Patients who have had a supracervical hysterectomy do not have improved sexual satisfaction or orgasm, nor are they less prone to develop pelvic organ prolapse (see Chapter Three) than a woman who has had a total hysterectomy. In fact, those who have undergone a SCH because of vaginal bleeding are more likely to report unwanted vaginal spotting months to years after the surgery. However, if you are having a specific type of surgery for prolapse called laparoscopic/robotic sacrocolpopexy, then a partial hysterectomy does have a medical advantage over a total hysterectomy (see Glossary of *Down There* Operations and/or Chapter Three for more details). On the other hand, if your cervix is not removed, then you will need to continue to have regular Pap smears. Regardless of these facts, some patients request SCH, and most doctors will honor their decision if they accept the associated risks and the necessity for regular surveillance for cervical cancer.

When You Need to Leave Your Uterus Alone

There are circumstances when a hysterectomy may be avoided. Although most cancers of the ovary, uterus, and cervix will require a hysterectomy, there are unique situations where a hysterectomy may not be required. In a young woman who has not had any children and who has a germ cell tumor on one of her ovaries, it is often possible to remove only the affected ovary without performing a hysterectomy or removing the other ovary. She will, however, require chemotherapy after the cancerous ovary has been removed. Additionally, for women who have not had children and who have nonaggressive cervical cancer, which has not spread to the lymph nodes, a surgery called radical trachalectomy can be an alternative solution. During this procedure, only the cervix and the surrounding tissues are removed, but the uterus is left intact. After this operation, two out of three women still can achieve pregnancy and deliver a baby; however, since the cervix is absent, a cerclage, or a purse-string suture, is wrapped around the lower part of the uterus, and a cesarean section will be necessary.

If a patient has pelvic organ prolapse and she doesn't want to have a hysterectomy, different surgical techniques can preserve the uterus while still fixing the prolapse. A uterine preserving technique for prolapse, which is a variation on sacrocolpopexy, is used to suspend the vagina, cervix, and uterus to the sacrum (see Chapter Three and Glossary of *Down There* Operations for more detail).

Wrapping it up

Regardless of all the alternatives mentioned above, the hysterectomy still is at the top of our list for achieving the best outcomes for our patients when the proper indications are met. For example, in a patient who is suffering from heavy vaginal bleeding, a hysterectomy has a 100 percent cure rate. Overwhelmingly, women who have considered all the above options, who make a well-informed choice to remove their uterus, and who have the surgery done by an experienced surgeon do very well. After a short period of recovery from the operation, our patients' quality of life improves after having a hysterectomy. For more advice on how best to recover after surgery see Chapter Twelve. Additionally, a credible website with good videos of what to expect before, during and after hysterectomy is www.hystersisters.com.

Let's return to Carolyn. During our interview with her, we had learned that her heavy bleeding had been occurring for more than a year. Every month, she bled so much that she got lightheaded and developed anemia (low red blood cell count). Because of her frequent bleeding and pain during intercourse, she had lost all interest in and desire for having sex with her husband.

Her previous doctor had treated Carolyn with birth control pills, and when this did not control the excessive bleeding, her doctor treated her with an intramuscular hormone shot (Depot Lupron). Neither one of these hormonal therapies had stopped her bleeding sufficiently, and she did not like the side effects of the Depot Lupron—the hot flashes, sweating, and irritability.

In considering a hysterectomy, Carolyn shared that she did not want to have any additional children. On our pelvic examination and with a pelvic ultrasound examination, we confirmed that her ovaries were normal, but that her uterus was enlarged with multiple fibroid tumors, which were the likely source of her abnormal heavy bleeding. We also reviewed her ultrasounds from years ago before she was being treated with hormones and found that her uterus showed a significant increase in size over several years.

Carolyn was worried about breast cancer because she recently had an abnormal mammogram; she revealed that her maternal grandmother had developed breast cancer at age 60. How did we advise Carolyn?

Due to her heavy bleeding and fibroids in multiple locations on her uterus, we felt that her body had not responded to conservative measures and that she was indeed a good candidate for surgery. The best options for her specific problems were either UAE or hysterectomy. Although a UAE might have improved or eliminated her symptoms, it would not provide a specimen to the pathologist to rule out cancer. Because the uterus had grown in size, Carolyn was worried about cancer in her uterus. After describing each of these procedures along with the pros and the cons, we came to the conclusion that hysterectomy was the best option for her.

The question remained whether Carolyn's ovaries should be removed. Since she didn't have a strong family history of breast cancer (despite her grandmother's cancer late in life), and her recent breast biopsy results were normal, the risks of removing her ovaries outweighed the benefits of removing them. At age 44, Carolyn's risk of dying from ovarian or breast cancer was less than the risk of having problems in the future related to osteoporosis and fracture, which could be more likely if the ovaries were removed at this age. Also, if we removed her ovaries at this age, she would go into menopause right away and have symptoms similar to side effects of Depot Lupron such as the hot flashes, sweating, and emotional upheaval.

We advised Carolyn to undergo a TVH and not to remove her ovaries. After we obtained proper consent by explaining the risks, benefits, and alternatives of a total vaginal hysterectomy and answering all of her questions, Carolyn chose to undergo TVH. During the surgery, her ovaries appeared normal (as was noted on ultrasound), and we did not remove them. She had a very quick recovery and was back to work in a month.

A pathologist examined her uterine tissue under a microscope, which indicated that it contained multiple fibroids and adenomyosis, which is a benign condition of uterine lining growing inside muscle, but there was no evidence of cancer of the uterus.

We've seen Carolyn every year for seven years, and she is very happy and healthy, and she states her sex life has improved since she is no longer worried about vaginal bleeding or pain. Her mammograms have also been normal.

Carolyn represents just one of our many happy patients, who—with good information and an explanation of all the benefits, risks, and potential problems that can occur—made an informed decision together with her doctor and has been happy after her hysterectomy.

The Bottom Line

If you are considering hysterectomy or have been recommended to have this procedure, it's important to keep in mind that a hysterectomy is safe and can alleviate your discomfort: if there are indications for it and if you've made an informed decision, then it can usually result in a happy ending.

Nearly half a million women each year are going to be confronted with the decision to have their uterus removed. This is not an easy decision to make. However, if you are knowledgeable about the procedure, understand the risks and complications, and know the alternatives, you and your gynecologist can come to a conclusion that will be safe, effective, and still preserve your femininity. This is a chapter you will want to read several times before meeting with your doctor and before pulling the trigger on your hysterectomy decision. So you see, even though something has to be removed down there, it can usually result in a happy ending!

Chapter Eleven

When You Want to Make It
Tighter and Prettier
Down There:
Vaginal Rejuvenation

Sylvia is a 49-year-old woman who had four children through vaginal deliveries while in her late twenties through her mid-thirties. Since that time, she noted that the looseness of her vagina became apparent during sexual intimacy and that she experienced less enjoyment during sex with her husband. As she said in a somewhat embarrassed voice, "Ever since I had my babies, I feel like I am too loose down there and don't please my husband anymore."

Before coming to see us, she had questioned her gynecologist, asking him, "Is there anything that you can do to help me?"

Like many gynecologists confronted with this situation, her doctor simply handed over a sheet of paper with instructions for Kegel exercises and told her, "You're a mom. There is nothing wrong with you and nothing you can do," and sent Sylvia on her way.

Let us be perfectly clear: vaginal rejuvenation surgery is controversial because no scientific studies have been published assessing the long-term satisfaction, safety, and complication rates for these procedures. Regardless of your opinion on this topic, what's important to know is that it's up to you. In Sylvia's case, her doctor was not thorough. He should have done a more complete exam, sent his patient to see a pelvic floor physical therapist (as we described in Chapter Five), or at the very least, explained to Sylvia how to make the Kegels more effective by doing the exercises correctly, more frequently, and regularly.

One afternoon, Sylvia happened to be watching a women-oriented talk show, and the hosts were discussing something she had never heard of—vaginal rejuvenation. This procedure was described as "plastic surgery" for the vagina. Sylvia was intrigued. Was it really possible to tighten the inside of her vagina so she could have more feeling during sex with her husband?

After seeing this show, Sylvia was curious enough—and frustrated enough with her own situation—to attend a seminar by one of the local gynecologists who performed these procedures. She had a laser vaginal rejuvenation or tightening procedure and, six weeks later, was able to engage in sexual intimacy with greater sexual gratification. It's important to note here that within the medical community, there are many anecdotal accounts of satisfaction with vaginal rejuvenation surgery, but as of yet, there are no significant studies that support statistically significant effectiveness; in fact, the doctor who patented this procedure will not allow research of laser vaginal rejuvenation. It's very important that if you are interested in having this procedure that you seek out a surgeon who is well qualified and has extensive experience in performing these procedures.

A Different Kind of Surgery

For decades, women have been flocking to plastic surgeons to have their wrinkles removed, their breasts augmented, their eyebrows lifted, and their tummies tucked. Now it is possible to apply those same principles of plastic surgery to the female parts down there. No one likes to have sagging, wrinkles or loss of function to any part of the body—even to those parts that aren't visible to the whole world. Indeed, the vagina, like any other compartment of the body, is not exempt from the impact of childbirth and aging. It, too, will show signs of loss of elasticity and tone, and weakening of the tissue, and will feel simply more loose.

Childbirth naturally and inevitably stretches the vaginal structures to allow the passage of the baby's head. This stretching results in weakening of the pelvic muscles, ligaments, and even the skin tissue of the outer vagina. This loss of ligament strength and muscle support for the pelvic structures is also a natural effect of aging—the older women become, the more they lose their elasticity in all tissue, from skin on the face, belly, arms, breasts, and yes, even the vagina. As we saw in Chapter Three, this loss of tissue tone can result in a prolapse, when the muscles around the opening of the vagina and supporting the walls of the vagina become weak and stretched out, allowing internal organs to bulge through. It is recommended that a gaping opening in the vagina also be repaired at the time of prolapse surgery and this is not considered cosmetic. However, even without prolapse, women can experience damage to the nerves supplying the vaginal canal as well as decreased friction in the vagina during sexual intimacy. Other women with less severe symptoms, like Sylvia, turn to these procedures simply to turn the vaginal clock backward and restore some of the tightness and tone to the area.

Sexologists have known since the classic work of Masters and Johnson in the 1960s that sexual gratification in the woman is in part related to the amount of friction that is generated by the penis during intercourse or with the use of a penis surrogate such as the woman's finger or a vibrator. When some women lose this aspect of their sexual experience, they may become frustrated and depressed. They miss the pleasure and sense of vitality that sex can bring. The concept of size in women is just the reverse of size in men. Men are always longing for wider, fatter, and longer penises. That's why every man looks to the right and left when he steps up to the urinal and compares the size of his penis to the person urinating in the urinal next to him. Men call this penis envy. However, large-sized, gaping vaginal openings are hardly the envy of most women.

The good news is that now both of these conditions, prolapse and vaginal looseness or relaxation, can be repaired. The two most popular procedures for vaginal rejuvenation are vaginoplasty, which is a tightening of the inside of the vagina (this procedure is also known as perineorrhaphy if done for medical reasons) and labiaplasty for the cosmetic repair of the outside the vagina, or the lips (a.k.a. labia).

What's going on down there is loss of vaginal tone, which is a result of weakness of the vaginal walls and the muscles in the pelvis that the walls are attached to. The vaginal canal is not a continuously open tube ready for sexual intimacy or the passage of a baby's head at the time birth. The vagina expands and becomes longer with stimulation. The depth of the vaginal opening is three to four inches but increases to five to seven inches when stimulated. According to Drs. John Miklos and Robert Moore, leading experts in vaginal reconstruction surgery, a healthy, well-toned vagina contributes to the pleasurable sensations of intercourse both at the area of the vaginal opening and deeper within the vaginal canal. When the vaginal walls become stretched or damaged or the muscles lose their tone, there is an increase in the diameter of the vaginal canal and vaginal opening. This stretching or damage may leave the vagina as a gaping organ rather than a compact, tight structure. When this occurs, it may also result in sagging or wrinkling of the labia. If the vaginal opening and canal are much looser and more relaxed than they were prior to childbirth, both the woman and her partner will more than likely experience a decrease in friction and a decrease in sensation and, ultimately, their enjoyment during intercourse.

This is exactly what Sylvia and her husband were experiencing, thus resulting in them looking into vaginal rejuvenation and fixing her problem down there.

Is This Procedure Right for You?

The most common symptom is decreased sensation or enjoyment during sexual intimacy. This symptom also includes decreased ability to achieve an orgasm during intimacy as a result of less friction between the erect penis and the vagina. If you have the sensation of vaginal looseness or relaxation at the opening of the vagina, this is strongly suggestive of laxity that can be remedied by vaginal rejuvenation. Certainly, Kegel exercises or pelvic floor muscle exercises should be attempted first prior to considering surgery. And again, you will probably make better progress if you do this with the help of a pelvic floor physical therapist or women's clinical specialist. However, if you have tried these exercises and they have not worked, then surgery may be an option. You can test the vaginal tension by gently inserting the index finger into the vagina. If the inserted finger can not sense a contraction of the vaginal muscles, then there may be a problem of vaginal looseness. Many women also note having to use larger tampons during their menstrual cycles, and even with larger ones, they find they move around or fall out. If the index finger test is inconclusive, then insert three fingers into the vaginal opening. If the three or more fingers fall into the vagina, this may be another sign of vaginal relaxation. (A rule of thumb for a proper-sized vaginal opening is if two fingers—usually the index and middle fingers—fit snugly in the vagina.)

Finally, if you find that you need to use larger and larger sex aids (i.e., vibrators) in order to achieve sexual gratification, then you may be experiencing vaginal relaxation.

Which Surgery Is Right for You?

Whether you are considering surgical options to either improve the appearance of your vagina (including the labia and clitoral hood), or to tighten and improve sexual functioning and gratification, there are a number of possible procedures available. Let's take a look at your options.

Vaginoplasty

A vaginoplasty procedure is the ideal choice to address the sagging or looseness of the vaginal canal and vaginal opening. Many women with grown children are now seeking rejuvenation of the vaginal tissues with the hope of enhancing the sexual experience for themselves and their mates. Vaginoplasty, sometimes referred to as rejuvenation of the vagina, is a procedure that can usually correct the problem of stretched vaginal walls resulting from childbirth(s) and is intended as a means of enhancing a woman's sexual life once again. The procedure typically repairs the stretched vaginal walls and tones the vaginal muscles, resulting in greater contraction strength and control, thereby permitting greater sensation during sexual experiences. Generally, anyone in average physical condition or good health can be a candidate for vaginoplasty surgery.

The purpose of the vaginoplasty is to reduce the caliber of the vaginal canal and opening of the vagina without sacrificing the vaginal length. The surgeon doesn't do a woman any favors by reducing the opening and shortening the length of the vagina—as a shortened vagina causes the penis to bump up against the cervix or the top of the vagina causing pain to both the woman and sometimes even to the man. Again, the goal of reconstructive vaginal surgery is to help create a long and appropriately narrow vagina—too narrow is bad because it causes pain with intercourse.

Incisions are created on the vaginal surface. A small amount of excess skin is removed, and the muscles at the opening of the vagina are brought together in the middle to return the vaginal canal and opening to its normal more youthful appearance. A laser or other high-energy cutting instrument is often used to reduce the bleeding during the procedure.

Vaginoplasty is usually done on an outpatient basis in a hospital or in a surgery center. The procedure is accomplished in less than an hour. Depending on the extent of the surgery, a vaginal pack may be inserted at the end of the procedure and is removed in the recovery room before you are discharged from the hospital. The tissue is usually injected with a local anesthetic, which reduces the pain after the procedure. The tissues are usually closed with absorbable sutures so no suture removal needs to occur in the postoperative period. Women are advised to avoid heavy lifting, strenuous exercise, or sexual intimacy for four to six weeks after the procedure. The doctor will give you the green light when you can resume sexual intimacy.

Labiaplasty

Just as the vagina is the passageway to the pleasure zone, the labia are the decorations on the doorway leading to the inside. The labia consist of a small set of vaginal tissue, or labia minora, and the larger set, or labia majora, which are external to the labia minora.

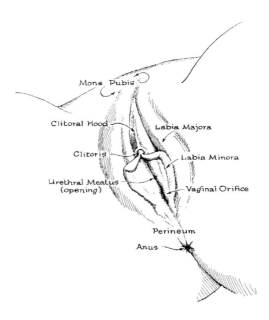

Some women find that floppy labia are a source of embarrassment when they undress—whether alone or in front of their partner. Some women even report a loss of self-esteem because they think oversized labia are a sexual turnoff. Women with this condition can also experience hygiene issues and irritation with simple everyday activities such as walking, wearing tight-fitting jeans, exercise, sports, toileting, wiping after bowel movement, and even pain and discomfort during intercourse. The labia may be very visible when a woman wears tight pants, swimsuits, or shorts making some women self-conscious about this. If a woman has a problem with large labia, or if one labia is larger than the other, a labiaplasty permits the reduction of large labia to reduce their outward appearance, to correct any irregularities, and to make everything symmetrical and smaller.

Labiaplasty can be done for either medical or aesthetic purposes. Medical reasons for labiaplasty (labia surgery) include the reduction of tissue from overly large or thick labia minora called labial hypertrophy that can result in constant irritation in tight pants and discomfort when engaging in sports or other physical activities. Overly large labia can also create discomfort and pain during intercourse as the labia are pulled into the vagina during penetration. In many of these instances, women are born with large labia—others may develop this condition with childbirth, age, friction, or as a result of an infection. Surgery of the labia represents a relatively safe solution for most medical reasons.

Aesthetic reasons (beautification) are largely being driven by societal evolution regarding women's rights and self-expression regarding sexual habits, wants, and expectations. Women now more than ever are able to have the freedom to express their feelings about sexuality, looks, and desire. This is one of the primary reasons driving the market for genital surgery and is chiefly responsible for the dramatic increase in labiaplasty, as women in everyday life are now demanding more options.

There are several options for the surgical reduction of the labia: direct labial contouring (linear excision), V-wedge resection, or Z-plasty procedure.

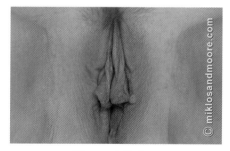
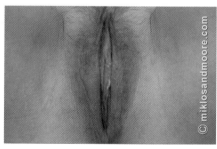

Figure 1 Before   Figure 2 After

* The authors wish to acknowledge Drs. John Miklos and Robert Moore (www.miklosandmoore.com), urogynecologists in Atlanta, Georgia, and the authors of *Vaginal Rejuvenation and Cosmetic Surgery of the Vulva and Vagina*. They are considered international experts in vaginal reconstruction and cosmetic vaginal surgery, and have graciously provided some content and allowed us to use the before and after photograph in this chapter.

Figure 1 shows a preoperative example of excessive labia, and Figure 2 shows the postoperative result after a labial contouring procedure. The V-wedge and the Z-plasty may be better to preserve the pigmentation on the edge of the labia minora. As of yet, there are no scientific studies that demonstrate that one procedure is superior to the other, so the choice usually comes down to the surgeon's preferences, recommendations, experiences, and the patients desired outcome.

Drs. Miklos and Moore, however, have noted that a majority of women notice a change or darkening in the edges of the labia when they enlarge. These women report that they do not like this discoloration, and they would like a return to the lighter or pinker edges they once had. This can only be done with linear contouring. Additionally, most women with enlarged labia also have extra skin folds around the clitoral hood called excess prepuce. These excess prepuce folds can also be reduced to achieve a natural cosmetic appearance. It takes an experienced surgeon to do this, so be sure to discuss this with your surgeon.

If the problem is caused by excess fat deposits in the labia majora, or the outer lips located on the outside of the labia minora, then this excess fatty tissue can be removed by liposuction to reduce the bulging in the area. However, in most cases, the enlarged labia majora is caused by excess skin; and in this case, the labia majora can also be reduced surgically by removing a wedge of excess skin and a small amount of underlying fat. Drs. Miklos and Moore inform their patients that surgery on the labia majora may result in a visible scar; however, many times the scars can be hidden in the folds between the labia majora and minora, and tiny absorbable sutures are used to minimize the scar formation.

Other women may desire the opposite effect when their labia majora become loose, saggy, or even wrinkled from a loss of fat deposit; these women may be motivated to make this area fuller, firmer, smoother and more youthful. These areas can be enhanced with the injection of collagen or using the women's own fat transferred from one area of the body to the labia. Middle-aged men and women know that most of us have some extra fat that can be easily spared from our waist and lower abdomens and transposed to areas that need to have a few wrinkles ironed out.

Labiaplasty is almost always an outpatient procedure performed under anesthesia. After surgery, patients may experience some mild discomfort and variable swelling, which usually disappears for the most part after one to two weeks. Recovery times range from three days to two weeks.

Most women can return to sexual intimacy in four to six weeks after the procedure.

It is normal to expect some bruising, swelling, and pain after the labiaplasty procedure. Some women describe the loss of sensation in the surgical areas treated. As the nerves begin to regenerate, feeling and sensation should return to normal. Swelling or firmness may linger for as long as several months.

Risks and Complications of Labiaplasty

Labiaplasty may require an additional treatment in 5 to 7 percent of cases just as other popular plastic surgical procedures, such as breast augmentation and liposuction, may require a second procedure or a revision.

Cutting-Edge Vaginal Rejuvenation Procedures

G-spot Amplification or G-shot

The elusive G-spot, a dime-size area typically found on the roof of the vagina, is often a source of sexual pleasure for women when stimulated. Some doctors believe that injecting this sensitive area with collagen increases a woman's sensitivity to stimulation. The collagen injection is done in the doctor's office under local anesthesia and takes just a few seconds. Unfortunately, the collagen is slowly absorbed, and the injection needs to be repeated every three to four months. Today, the medical community raises an eyebrow as to the effectiveness of this procedure, as there are no studies to prove that the procedure actually works. Nevertheless, patients ask for it, and some doctors are happy to give it.

Anal Bleaching

Anal bleaching (or anal lightening) is the process of bleaching the darker pigmentation around the anus. Melanin is a chemical naturally produced by our bodies, which darkens skin color. The more melanin produced, the darker the skin. The procedure is accomplished by the application of a topical cream usually containing hydroquinone to the anus. Other chemicals used to bleach the anal area contain mercury. These chemicals have been implicated in causing cancer and have been banned in the United Kingdom and France. Anal bleaching can also cause chemical burns to a very sensitive area.

Women do anal bleaching for strictly cosmetic purposes, and to tell you the truth, as doctors, we are not sure what motivates a woman to make a decision to bleach this area. Adult film stars have used anal bleaching to provide a less pigmented appearance of the area so that the anus is similar in appearance to the surrounding skin. But since beauty is in the eye of the beholder, we aren't passing judgment on those who wish to pursue this course of action.

Hymenoplasty

The name hymen is derived from the Greek god of marriage, Hymen, and has been a mark of virginity since the beginning of time. The hymen is a ringlike skin membrane that sits in the opening of the vagina. Most often there is a five-or six-pointed star opening in the hymen after maturity. However, there are multiple formations of hymens that can be present at birth. A few of these configurations are shown in the illustration on the next page. The septate and microperforate hymens may be incompatible with sexual intercourse if the remaining hymenal tissue is thick. The imperforate hymen is incompatible with sex or the ability to have regular menstrual periods and must be incised.

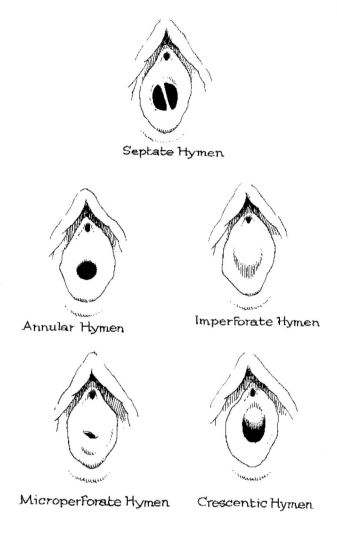

Septate Hymen

Annular Hymen

Imperforate Hymen

Microperforate Hymen

Crescentic Hymen

It is widely known and accepted that the hymen can be ruptured by nonsexual activity, such as dancing, horseback riding, athletics, or the use of tampons. At one time, a bride's hymen being intact was the only way to determine her chastity. In the past, midwives were known to disguise a broken hymen by sewing it up with a needle and thread, at times using the membrane material of sheep, goats, and other animals.

If the hymen has been torn by sexual intimacy or by nonsexual activity, it can be reconstructed as if nothing ever occurred. Hymen repair or hymenoplasty is usually done at the request of someone who needs the surgery for ethnic, cultural, or religious reasons.

This procedure is more popular in the Middle East and in Latin America where there is a premium for women to be virgins at the time of marriage. This revirginization is performed in an effort to appease religious, cultural, and societal beliefs. Women may seek it out prior to their wedding to make their future mother-in-law and perhaps their husband convinced that they have never had sexual intimacy. If the surgery goes as planned, the hymen will tear and will cause pain and a small amount of blood loss. Now the mother of the bride can parade the soiled sheets to all concerned, and the couple can live happily ever after.

The hymenoplasty is usually done in the doctor's office under local anesthesia. Small dissolvable stitches are used to reconnect the skin membrane that once partially covered the opening to the vagina. Recovery time is about six weeks.

Clitoral Unhooding (Hoodectomy)

Clitoral unhooding, also referred to as hoodectomy, is a minor feminine genital surgical procedure to remove excess tissue or the surrounding hood that covers the clitoris. Normally, the prepuce or hood is anatomically designed to offer the clitoris a degree of protection against undue friction or abrasion or over stimulation. The clitoral hood naturally retracts during sexual intercourse—thereby leaving the highly innervated surface of the clitoris to be more exposed resulting in female sexual orgasms. Sometimes, however, women with small clitoral nodes or those that have excess prepuce tissue find that they can't achieve orgasm, or have a harder time reaching climax, because the clitoris is literally covered, or restricted by too much skin tissue, thus greatly lessening tactile sensation, and/or even eliminating it entirely.

Clitoral unhooding is sometimes referred to as female clitoral circumcision as the procedure is somewhat analogous to penile circumcision in men. This is to be differentiated and separated from the highly controversial, de-feminizing procedure of female circumcision, in which some or all parts of the clitoris, labia minora, and labia majora are removed. Female circumcision takes place in certain African countries. Hoodectomy is nowhere in the ballpark of female circumcision. In the United States, hoodectomy is done more commonly to allow women to experience heightened arousal, by reducing the tissue that forms the hood or covering of the clitoris. To some extent, it has been suspected that excessive prepuce tissue can also result in some hygiene-related issues as well for women, giving sanctuary to harmful bacteria, and sometimes resulting in what are commonly termed yeast or vaginal infections from the close proximity of the clitoris to the vaginal canal.

The Bottom Line

Many women and men want to turn back the biologic clock and have a more youthful appearance. Although plastic surgery on the face and breasts offers more visible results, vaginal rejuvenation procedures also attempt to provide women with a more youthful vagina. The results may help women increase their self-esteem, their confidence, and may enhance the sexual pleasure for themselves and for their partners. Who could ask for anything more?

Chapter Twelve

What You Want to Know
Before and After Having Surgery
Down There:
Pre-and Postoperative Care

There's probably no bigger decision you will ever make than to have elective pelvic surgery. This is not a decision to take lightly. What you do to prepare for this event will have a significant impact on how well you do before, during, and after the surgery. For the most part, we are all out of our comfort zone when we submit to undergoing a surgical procedure. We will turn over every aspect of our life, including our breathing, to doctors who will do everything they can to ensure that all goes well, but there are always a number of unknowns that any person confronts. The more of these unknowns that you are able to anticipate, the more likely you will reduce the anxiety that comes before surgery and speed up your recovery after surgery.

This chapter will help you to better understand the concept of elective surgery and what you can expect before the procedure and what you need to know after the procedure. We will provide you with checklists that you can use in preparation and other tips on how to set yourself up for a very smooth pre and postoperative experience.

Unfortunately, doctors and their nurses don't always spend the time with patients to prepare them for surgery. Doctors or the staff will often go over the surgical consent with the patient and provide the patient with educational material about the procedure or direct her to the Internet for credible websites that describe the procedure in greater detail. It is no wonder that patients are often confused, anxious, or even frightened about elective surgery.

What to Expect

Surgery isn't just making an incision, removing or repairing a diseased organ, and then closing the skin. You will need to be prepared both physically, mentally, emotionally, and even spiritually. The more preparation you have taken, the better your outcome will be and the lower the level of discomfort you will experience after the procedure. The more knowledge you have about the procedure and know what to expect, the less anxiety you will experience; this means you will endure less emotional trauma after the procedure.

Today, most of the surgical procedures described in this book are done in one-day surgical centers or ambulatory surgery centers. This means you will go to the hospital days or weeks before the procedure for your preoperative preparation. At that time, you will become familiar with the surgery center, meet the nurses and technicians who will be caring for you, and have an interview with the anesthesiologist, the doctor who will be giving you the anesthesia or putting you to sleep. If you are going to an ambulatory or a one-day surgical center, you will be told when to arrive, which is usually several hours before the procedure; you will have the surgery and then be discharged when you are medically stable. This means your blood pressure is normal, you have tolerated a liquid diet, you are able to urinate, the pain is controlled, and you are able to walk around without dizziness.

Some of these procedures can be done under sedation or using local anesthesia. As a result of the shorter operating times, the incisions are confined to the vagina or lower abdomen, resulting in less postoperative problems and complications.

Emergency Surgery vs. Elective Surgery

Emergency surgery is usually necessary after an injury or if there is medical situation that needs immediate attention. There is no planning for emergency surgery. You need it right away, and you don't have any decisions to make. You often don't select your surgeon, your hospital, or your anesthetic. On the other hand, elective surgery is a decision you must make for yourself. You have to decide if the procedure is worth the risks; and if not having surgery is the option you wish to choose, then accept that the problem will not take care of itself and may even become worse if surgery is avoided.

Selecting the Right Hospital

You may have a choice about where to have your surgery, since most doctors can operate at several hospitals/surgery centers. A good first step is to ask your doctor which facilities he/she uses and which he/she prefers. You also want to be sure that the facility has experience with the procedure. It is well accepted that facilities that perform a large number of a particular procedure, in excess of eight to ten a month, have better outcomes than facilities that only rarely perform a procedure. Just imagine a wedding planner that does several dozen weddings a year and compare his/her skills to a wedding planner that does two weddings a year and one of them wasn't the royal wedding of Kate Middleton and Prince William!

Which one would you imagine would do a better job for you or your daughter? The same applies to your selection of a hospital or ambulatory treatment center. Those facilities that do more procedures have an operating room and nursing staff that are familiar with the instruments and equipment needed for the procedure. Their familiarity will help the surgeon, and anesthesiologist make your procedure proceed without hitches or delays. Also, a nursing staff that is familiar with the procedure can help answer any unanswered questions before your procedure and help with your postoperative recovery. Obtaining information about the volume of cases performed at a facility may be a little difficult. You can call the facility and ask to speak to the director of the operating room or you can call the hospital public relations department and ask for information, which they will usually share with you.

It has been the tradition for the doctor and the practice to tell the patient the date and time that the procedure is scheduled. However, this age-old tradition is changing. Today, it is definitely appropriate for a patient to be more assertive and provide a few dates that are convenient for her and ask the doctor's scheduler to make the surgical date that is convenient for both the doctor and patient.

A Healthy Body Means a Quick Recovery

Your heart and lungs are vital to your surgical success. You want to be in good shape for your big day. This means you want to be in tiptop cardiovascular shape. If you are not already involved in a regular exercise program, you may want to consider becoming more active several months in advance of your surgery. Walking, jogging, and swimming are all helpful in getting you into good physical shape.

If you are a smoker, right now would be a good time to quit. Smoking hinders the transfer of oxygen from the air you breathe into the circulation to be carried to all the tissues. If you are a smoker, your heart and lungs will work harder to get oxygen to your tissues during and after surgery and can retard the healing process. Word of advice: if you're going to stop smoking, it is better to do it few weeks (four or more) before surgery as stopping smoking a few days before surgery can do more harm than good!

Your calorie consumption is also vital to the surgery and the healing process. It is probably not a good idea to go on a diet and reduce your caloric consumption before surgery. However, it is important to eat a diet that is high in fiber and protein before surgery. It is also helpful to decrease your consumption of empty calories—so cut back on white sugar, processed foods, and any foods that are high in sodium or fat.

Your doctor will certainly have taken a careful history of your previous medical conditions and also be knowledgeable about your medications and allergies. It is imperative to reveal to your doctor all the medications that you take including over-the-counter drugs, herbals, and supplements. If you have risk factors for surgery such as previous heart attack, stroke, or heart failure, then your doctor will give you a medication called a beta-blocker to reduce your chance of having a serious heart problem during and after surgery.

Other medications and herbals, such as kava kava and *Ginkgo biloba*, can interact with drugs that you might receive before, during, or after the procedure. If you are taking these supplements or over-the-counter medications, you should discuss with your doctor when you should stop the medication and when you can start taking the medications after your procedure. Also, it is necessary to discuss the management of any blood thinners you may be taking such as aspirin, warfarin (Coumadin), or Plavix (see the box below for a list of common medications that thin your blood).

Blood Thinners That Should Be Stopped Prior to Major Surgery

Aspirin (Bayer, Ecotrin, others)

Mobic (meloxicam)

Clopidogrel (Plavix)—stop five days

Arthritis medications—Arthrotec, etc.

Dipyridamole (Persantine)

Motrin, Advil (ibuprofen)

Pletal

Ticlopidine (Ticlid)—stop two weeks

Piroxicam (Feldene, Fexicam)

Eptifibatide (Integrilin)

Naprosyn, Alleve (naproxen)

Celebrex or Bextra

Nambumeton (Relafen)

Sulindac (clinoril)

Tirofiban (aggrastat)

Coumadin*

Vitamin E

Fish oil

*Ask your doctor if you should be switched to heparin or Lovenox before discontinuing Coumadin.

Additionally, you should stop taking the four Gs (ginger, garlic, ginko, and ginseng) at least a week before surgery as they can also thin your blood and increase your risk of bleeding. The box below lists common herbs and supplements that may interfere with anticoagulant medications and may make you susceptible to bleeding during surgery.

Common Herbs and Supplements that Can Interact with Other Medications and Cause Bleeding

Garlic
Ginger
Gingko
Ginseng
Fish oil
St. John's wort
Glucosamine-chondroitin
Grapefruit juice
Coenzyme Q10
Cranberry juice
Curbicin
Chinese wolfberry
Dong quai
Fenugreek
Green tea
Melatonin
Omega-3
Papaya extract
Quilinggao

Doctors have different opinions about over-the-counter pain medications such as Advil, ibuprofen, and Aleve. For minor procedures such as a biopsy, your doctor may permit these minor pain relievers before surgery. In each case, you need to discuss this with your doctor and certainly advise him/her of your use of these medications.

Many women use medications to control blood pressure, to treat diabetes, and to help control depression. Your doctor or the anesthesiologist may allow you to take these medications with a sip of water before the surgery. If you take insulin for diabetes, you may be instructed to adjust the dosage since you will not be taking any food for several hours. Again, a discussion with the doctor or the anesthesiologist is in order.

The Night Before

You will probably be asked to avoid any food or fluids after midnight before surgery. An anaesthetic may relax the muscles in the stomach and esophagus, the tube between the mouth and the stomach, and result in the stomach contents regurgitating and ending up in the lungs. This can lead to pneumonia, which is a serious condition requiring hospital admission. Therefore, it is very important to keep the stomach empty, and this can best be accomplished by stopping food and fluids the night before the procedure. Be sure to adhere to this request as having food in your stomach may delay or even result in cancellation of your surgery. If your surgery is later in the day, then check with your doctor or the nurse, as you may be able to have a clear liquid breakfast.

You may be asked to take a laxative or an enema the night before or the morning of your surgery. The purpose of the enema is to empty the rectum of stool as most women become constipated after surgery. Constipation is common because women are not as active after the procedure and also the use of pain medication can promote constipation. Therefore, it is better to have an empty colon and rectum before your surgical procedure. An empty rectum is also helpful for your surgeon who is performing urogynecologic and pelvic surgery.

You will probably be given prescriptions for medications to take after surgery. These may include pain medication, antibiotics, and medications to avoid constipation. If possible, we suggest that you have these medications filled prior to your procedure. You don't want to come home from the hospital and experience pain and not have any medication readily available.

We also strongly recommend that you do not help the surgeon and start the surgery by shaving the night before the procedure. Usually shaving can result in small cuts or abrasions in the skin, and this can be a source of a postoperative infection. We do suggest that you take a shower using one of the over-the-counter antibacterial soaps the day before surgery to reduce infection risk. Examples of antibacterial soaps include Cuticura Medicated

Anti-Bacterial Bar Soap, Safeguard Antibacterial Bar Soap with Aloe, and Cetaphil Antibacterial Gentle Cleansing Bar.

Questions for the Doctor:

When should I return for an appointment after surgery?
When should I change the dressing?
Anything special I need to know about the incision?
Are my stitches absorbable, or do they need to be removed?
When can I return to work? Lifting? Exercise? Douching? Sexual intimacy?
When can I shower? Bath? Jacuzzi?
When and what can I eat?
When should I call the doctor?
What medications will I need after the surgery?
When can I resume my regular medications after surgery?
If I use aspirin or other blood thinners, when can I start the medication after surgery?
Do I need to take a blood thinner for a short period of time after surgery?
Who do I call if I have an emergency?

What to Bring to the Hospital:

Insurance information
Driver's license or photo ID
Loose-fitting clothing to wear after your procedure
Comfortable shoes—not shoes that have laces
Toothbrush and toothpaste
Instructions or orders from your doctor
Consent from the doctor's office
A container to place your dentures or dental plate in
A list of all of your medications
Advance directives if you have a living will
Arrange transportation from the hospital as you will not
    be allowed to drive home after you receive an anesthetic

What Not to Bring
    Do not wear or bring makeup
    Do not wear or bring contact lenses
    Do not bring money, jewelry, or valuables

Getting Your Mind Ready for the Surgery

Putting your body in the ready is only half of the preparation. The other segment, the mind, is every bit as important. What you can do to be in the right frame of mind before surgery will significantly impact your experience in the hospital or treatment center and how quickly you can resume all normal activities.

We recommend a book and CD, *Prepare for Surgery, Heal Faster* by Peggy Huddleston. This book nicely illuminates what you should do to prepare your mental attitude for the surgery. We will summarize these five steps:

Step 1. Relaxation: The first step involves learning how to relax and get around your fears and terrors about surgery. Peggy teaches a deep relaxation skill to be practiced before surgery and afterward (which can be useful throughout life). As many of you know already, deep relaxation may bring up some unexpected emotions. All of us carry around some unresolved tension and stress, and this experience is a good one for letting that all come out. Deep relaxation can improve your immune system. This can make a huge difference in recovery from surgery. Peggy recommends listening to her audio recording (or there are others) for 30 minutes each day for two weeks before surgery for optimal benefit.

Step 2. Visualization: The second step adds to relaxation by envisioning your healing. Imagine yourself feeling good, comfortable, and happy after the operation will go a long way toward creating that very result. Her studies also show that seeing yourself surrounded by a healing light, sound, or a sense of deep peace can be very powerful. Again, to repeat this visualization every day with the relaxation exercises is the most beneficial. You can even bring the tapes, CDs, or now your iPod into the operating room, and play them during your procedure.

Step 3. Support: In the third step, you are encouraged to ask for help. You can create a network of friends, relatives, or coworkers to be your team, assigning them particular duties or times to help you—before surgery, during, or afterward—to visit you, assist at home, take care of the kids, or whatever else needs to be done. One interesting request that some of our patients report as helpful is to have your team envision you on a pink healing cloud the day of your surgery, and to send more such clouds to you throughout the healing process.

Step 4. Healing words: The next step involves giving a list of healing statements to be spoken by the surgeon or anesthesiologist before and after your surgery. The first is, "Following this operation, you will feel comfortable, and you will heal very well." The next are open-ended statements to be completed by the patient, including: "Following this operation, you will be hungry for_____"; now insert your wish, and the doctor will give you this postanesthetic suggestion. Now we can't tell you that this always works, but we can certainly say with unequivocal certainty that it won't hurt!

Step 5. A meeting: The final step in Peggy's book is to meet with your anesthesiologist prior to surgery. This is often the most difficult step because it is simply difficult to arrange. Preop clinics are supervised by doctors who will most likely not be the particular anesthesiologist doing your case. But you can tell them that you are preparing for your surgery, and they should note that on your chart. This is the time to review your past experiences with anesthesia (if you have had them), and how you would like to feel afterward.

If you are still feeling terrified of having surgery after going through the five steps and can't relax or get peaceful about it, Peggy Huddleston also offers phone consults. She is available at (800) 726-4173. Alternatively, she may be able to recommend someone in your community who has undergone her training.

S-Day (Surgery Day)

You will arrive at the hospital or treatment center several hours before your procedure. A nurse will take you to a preoperative room where all the preparation will take place. The nurse will check your records and orders, and be sure that your consent has been properly signed and dated. Usually the nurse will ask you questions about the name of the procedure you are going to have, the name of your doctor, and your medications and allergies. You will be given an identification bracelet that has your name, date of birth, and hospital identification number. It is a good idea to look at the bracelet and be certain that all the information is correct. You will then remove your clothing and change into one of those less-than-flattering hospital gowns that were developed decades ago and haven't been modified to protect a woman's dignity or comfort. The gowns are created not for the ballroom but for the operating room so as to have easy access to the surgical site and to easily be removed in the operating room once the anesthetic has been administered. The nurse will then start an intravenous line, or IV. This is how fluids and medications are given to you during the procedure. A blood pressure cuff will be placed on the opposite arm from the IV. Your blood pressure will be taken in the preoperative area and monitored the entire time you are having your procedure.

If you have dentures, you will be asked to remove them and place them into a container that has your name and identification numbers. If you have caps on your teeth, especially your front teeth, be sure to tell the nurse and the anesthesiologist as special precautions will be taken not to injure your teeth.

You will also be asked to remove eyeglasses, jewelry, and hearing aids before going to the operating room. Depending upon the surgery, you may be given tight-fitting stockings that go from your toes to your mid thigh. These stocking are used to compress the veins and reduce the risk of blood clots forming in your legs. Now there are calf pumps that can be worn around the calves that intermittently fill with air to compress and massage the blood vessels and prevent blood from clotting in the veins in your lower legs.

Just before you are leaving the preoperative area, the anesthesiologist or a nurse anesthetist will come into the room and identify himself or herself and ask you the very same questions the nurse asked you when you were admitted to the preoperative area. The doctor does all these checks to be absolutely certain that the right patient receives the right operation and on the right area. At this time, you can give and receive a hug from your family member and/or friend, and the nurse anesthetist will administer a sedative that will make you sleepy but not put you to sleep. A nurse anesthetist from the preoperative staging area will then transport you on a gurney or a stretcher to the operating room.

Once you are in the operating room, you will be asked to move from the stretcher to the operating room table. The nurses and aides will help assist you in moving to the operating table. Once you are on the operating table, a comfortable strap will be placed around your abdomen to be certain that you do not fall from the operating room table.

Most patients are sedated when they enter the operating room, but for those who are awake and want to look around, you will be amazed at what you see. There will be huge operating room lights, large pieces of equipment that will monitor your heart rate, blood pressure and the amount of oxygen in your bloodstream. You may see a number of computer screens that will display what the surgeon is seeing during your procedure especially if you are having a laparoscopic surgery and the tiny camera is attached to one of the instruments that is inserted through a pencil-sized opening in your abdomen. You may see four to six people scurrying around with masks and surgical hats as they prepare the instruments that your doctor will be using. You might feel the same awe that you experience when you walk onto an airplane and look at all the controls and dials that are in the cockpit that make it possible to fly the plane.

The operating room is kept a little colder than what you are used to (around 69°F). This is because the doctors and nurses wear gowns and gloves and can get warm during the surgery. But don't worry—you will be covered with heated blankets to be sure that you don't become cold.

In our operating room, we like to play soothing music just before and throughout your surgery. We believe this not only helps the surgeon and staff in the operating room to remain calm and focused, but it also subconsciously may have a positive effect on you during surgery.

Often, the nurse anesthetist will hook up all the equipment in preparation for the anesthesiologist to come and administer the anesthetic that truly puts you to sleep. Usually a mask will be placed over your nose and mouth, and you will be given oxygen to breathe before the intravenous anesthetic is given and the tube inserted that will give you the oxygen and the anesthetic gases that keep you asleep during the surgery.

This is a very orchestrated series of events. However, if you know what to expect and are prepared, you will relax and may even enjoy the deepest sleep you ever had. Think about your favorite place in the world as you go off to sleep.

After the Surgery Is Over

What you do after surgery is just as important to the overall success of your operation as what happens before and during surgery. Postoperative care begins the moment you are moved from the operating table to the gurney that transports you to the recovery room.

Postoperative recovery starts in the postanesthesia care unit, or PACU, the area where you will remain until you are fully awake and can return to the one-day-stay area or are admitted to a hospital room if your surgery is more extensive and you are going to have a longer recovery period.

Although it may take only seconds to receive anesthesia and go into a deep sleep, recovery from anesthesia takes time. It takes time for the anesthesia to be eliminated from the body's tissues. Many factors affect the amount of time a patient may spend in the recovery room. These factors include the preoperative medication, the type of anesthetic used, the length of time an anesthetic was administered during the surgery, your body's fat content, how you respond to these medications, and your tolerance to pain.

In the PACU, you will be in a cubicle or separated from the next patient by a curtain. Computers and monitors that will provide the nurses the important vital signs such as your temperature, pulse, blood pressure, respirations, and the amount of oxygen in your bloodstream will again surround you.

The recovery room nurses will usually speak to you in a low, reassuring voice and let you know what they are doing such as taking your blood pressure, checking your dressing, and perhaps checking the output from any tubes or catheters that are inserted at the time of surgery.

If you had an operation for pelvic organ prolapse, you will have some packing inside your vagina, which will be removed the next morning. You will also have an IV in place that provides you with fluids until you are able to start drinking water and other clear liquids. It is not uncommon to feel cold in the recovery room, and the nurses will place warm blankets on top of your covers to bring your body temperature to normal.

The nurses in the recovery room will encourage you to take a deep breath periodically and will help you sit up and take deep breaths and cough, which will clear your lungs of the secretions and anesthetic gases that may have accumulated during surgery.

If you have a long operation or are elderly, you may have compression devices on your lower legs. These compression devices fill with air every few minutes to simulate the effect of walking and moving the blood from the lower extremities back into circulation. They feel like leg massagers and are used to prevent deep vein thrombosis (DVT), where blood remains stagnant in the lower extremities and can clot and then travel to other parts of the body.

Nearly every hospital or surgery center has criteria that needs to be met before discharge will take place. For pelvic surgery, this usually means stable vital signs. The rule of thumb is that the vital signs have to be within 20 points of the preoperative vital signs. For example, if your blood pressure before the surgery is 120/80, then the blood pressure has to be 100-140/60-100. Or if your pulse is 80 before surgery, you can be discharged if your pulse is between 60 and 100. Again, these are rules of thumb and not carved in stone. If you had outpatient surgery, you have to demonstrate that you can tolerate fluids. Once you can do that, the IV line will be removed. You will want to be sure that the pain is under control and that you can be managed on oral medications at home. Also, you have to be able to walk, albeit slowly, from the bed to a chair or with the assistance of a nurse or your own caregiver. Lastly, the nurse will examine the incision and the dressing to be sure that there is no bleeding or drainage from the incision. Once you have met these milestones, you will be asked to sign a form and then can be discharged from the hospital. Since you have had an anesthetic, you will not be able to drive yourself home and will need a ride from the hospital to your home.

Catheter

Approximately 20% of women who have vaginal surgery will have some minor difficulty urinating after the surgery such as burning on urination or going to the restroom frequently. Only a few will develop urinary retention or inability to urinate. Most women will be given a trial of voiding if a catheter was inserted at the time of surgery. The trial of voiding consists of filling the bladder with water then removing the catheter and allowing the woman to try and urinate. If she is unable to urinate, the catheter will be reinserted and the catheter is attached to a leg bag or a larger bag that can attach to the clothing or to the bed. Now when the bag fills with urine, the bag has a drainage tube that can be opened and emptied into a container or the toilet. This prevents urine from accumulating in the bladder but drains to the outside of the body into the bag. Alternatively, your doctor may want you to plug-and-release the catheter. With this method, when you get the urge to urinate, you unplug the catheter and allow your bladder to empty and then plug the catheter when you're done.

Depending upon the nature of the surgery, the doctor will remove the catheter immediately before you go home or up to 7 days after surgery in the office, or in some cases the patient will remove the catheter herself, which is easy to do. If the woman is still unable to urinate after one week, a decision will be made to reinsert the catheter for a few more days or to teach the woman how to catheterize herself. The latter is referred to as intermittent catheterization and consists of a straw-size clean catheter that is easily inserted through the urethra into the bladder to drain the bladder of urine and then is removed and thrown away. Intermittent catheterization is usually done every 4-6 hours and especially before going to bed and upon awakening in the morning.

Nearly all women will be able to return to normal urination in a few days after starting a program of intermittent catherization or having the Foley catheter reinserted. Rarely will a woman not be able to urinate after surgery; and if this occurs your doctor may suspect an underlying neurological problem such as long-standing diabetes. Most women with these conditions will have bladder testing before the surgery and the doctor can predict if permanent urinary retention may be a possibility.

Pain Management After Your Surgery

Every operation creates some lingering pain. Pain is usually greater following an abdominal operation where an incision is made. Less pain occurs after laparoscopic or vaginal surgery. Fortunately, medications are helpful in alleviating pain and discomfort after surgery.

Recovery room nurses will ask if you are having any pain. They will record your response on a scale of 1-10 and provide you with pain medication as considered appropriate. A few minutes later, the nurses will ask you again about your pain level and give you additional medication if needed until the pain is under control. The effects of the anesthesia persist after surgery, providing an extended relief from pain in the immediate postoperative period. Also, surgeons commonly inject a local anesthetic in the incisions that will reduce the pain for several hours after the procedure.

In the recovery room, you may be offered an injection of pain medication, such as Dilaudid, morphine, or other opioids. If you are a candidate, we also prefer to give Toradol intravenously; this medication reduces the amount of narcotics you need when you awaken from the anaesthetic and helps with both pain and inflammation. Once you have started taking fluids by mouth, you may be switched to an oral pain medication such as Percocet or Norco.

For patients who are going to be admitted to the hospital, they may have access to patient-controlled anesthesia (PCA). This is a very sophisticated method of allowing the patient to control when she receives the pain medication. PCA refers to an electronically controlled infusion pump that delivers a set, small amount of IV analgesic (usually an opioid) that is controlled by the patient. This device is very appreciated by the patient, as you won't have to hit the call button for the nurse and wait for the medication to relieve your pain. When you feel the pain starting to increase, you just press the PCA button, and pain relief is just moments away. Because it is preset, the patient cannot overuse the medication. Some patients use the PCA for just a day or two after the procedure and then are converted to oral medication for pain control. PCA is usually used after abdominal operations.

You will also be provided with pain medication when you go home. You can use the stronger pain pills for a few days, and then consider using the medication only at night for sleeping and a milder painkiller, like

Motrin or Tylenol, during the day. Be sure to tell your doctor as well as the anesthesiologist before your surgery if you have any special circumstances or sensitivities to pain medication.

Food and Fluids

Some patients experience nausea after surgery, which is why the first thing you will be offered for several hours after surgery is a few ice chips, a few sips of water, or clear liquids. During this time, your nutrition needs will be met through the intravenous fluids. You will then progress from clear liquids to a regular diet.

Your diet after surgery is very important. You should make an effort to eat a balanced diet of protein, carbohydrates, and minimal fats. You should eat plenty of fresh fruits and vegetables to add fiber to your diet. You should also consider the use of a multivitamin that contains calcium and vitamin D.

Constipation is a common problem following surgery because of the decrease in motility of your bowels as well as pain medications (especially the opioids) that also promote constipation. But don't worry, the constipation can be managed by increasing the fiber in the diet, getting on your feet and walking soon after the operation, and using stool softeners, such as Colace or Dulcolax tablets or suppositories, and osmotic laxitives such as Lactulose. Also, good old water is medicinal and will help with constipation. So drink plenty of fluids after surgery. And don't forget about walking!

If these steps do not work, then stimulant laxatives such as bisacodyl cascara or an enema may be necessary. Be sure to tell your doctor if you are prone to constipation before your surgery, and steps can be taken to alleviate or eliminate this problem. On the next few pages, we have listed a remedy, delicious recipes, as well as some basic tips to help you keep constipation at bay.

Managing constipation after your surgery

More than 10% of woman are plagued with constipation for days to weeks after pelvic surgery. The vast majority of all patients suffering from constipation respond well to conservative therapies including changes in diet and use of mild laxatives. Here are four tips to help you move your bowels:

1. increase physical activity and light exercise to improve peristalsis, or squeezing movement of the intestines
2. increasing fluid intake—about 8 cups of fluid for a woman weighing 130 pounds, and more or less depending on your weight and activity level.
3. you might also consider adding a mild non-prescription laxative such as MiraLAX® to help make the stool more spongy. This can be take every day and is safe.
4. increase dietary fiber (30-35 grams per day) and even fiber supplements, especially insoluble fiber (such as psylium) that adds bulk and weight to the stool. In the box below we have included three high-fiber, great-tasting recipes from the National Association For Continence (www.nafc.org):

Special Remedy

> 1 cup applesauce
> 1 cup oat bran
> 1/4 cup prune juice
> Spices as desired (cinnamon, nutmeg, etc.)

This recipe may be stored in your refrigerator or in the freezer. Pre-measured servings may be frozen in sectioned ice cube trays, or foam plastic egg cartons, and thawed as needed.

Begin with two tablespoons each evening followed by one 6 to 8 ounce glass of water or juice. After 7 to 10 days increase this to three tablespoons. At the end of the second to third week increase it to four tablespoons. You should begin to see an improvement in your bowel habits in two weeks. You should make this a part of your daily routine for your lifetime. It is good for you!

When you begin using the Special Recipe, remember it is high fiber. You may be troubled by gas and bloating, but this should go away in several weeks.

Spring Vegetable Pesto Pasta

- 8 cloves garlic
- 1/3 cup pine nuts
- ¾ lb. whole wheat fusilli or pene pasta
- 1 lb. thin asparagus spears, trimmed and cut into 2" pieces
- 2 cups peas, fresh, or thawed from frozen, divided
- 6 oz. basil, stems discarded (about 5 cups loosely packed)
- 8 sprigs mint, stems discarded (about 1 cup loosely packed)
- 1 oz. freshly grated Parmesan (1/2-3/4 cup depending on the grater)
- ¼ cup extra-virgin olive oil
- Freshly ground black pepper
- 1 tsp kosher salt, divided

Preheat the oven to 300 degrees F. Lightly brush or spray the garlic with oil. Roast the garlic with the pine nuts on a baking sheet until the nuts are golden brown and the garlic has softened, about 12 minutes. Boil the pasta in large pot of water. Add the asparagus 2 minutes before the pasta is finished cooking. Add 1 ½ cups of peas when the pasta is done. Turn off the burner, drain the pasta and vegetables, and return them to the pot. Now make pesto. In a food processor, pulse the roasted garlic and pine nuts with the basil, mint, ½ cup of peas, half of the Parmesan, and the oil until uniformly chopped. Season with pepper and ½ tsp of salt. Scoop out ½ cup of pasta water and stir it into pesto. Toss the pasta and vegetables with the pesto. Serve immediately sprinkled with the remaining ½ tsp. of salt and the remaining Parmesan. Serves 4.1

Per Serving (2 ½ cups) *Calories: 480 Sodium: 500 mg Total Fat: 19g Cholesterol: 10 mg Sat. Fat: 3.5g Carbohydrates: 65g Protein: 20g Fiber 12g*

Curried Lentils

- 1 cup green or French lentils
- 1 carrot, peeled and diced
- ¼ cup canola oil
- 1 onion, diced
- 4 cloves garlic, minced
- 1 Tbs grated ginger
- 1 Tbs. curry powder
- 1 tsp turmeric (optional)
- 1 15 oz can of no-salt-added diced tomatoes
- 2 unpeeled apples, cored and diced
- ½ cup whole milk plain yogurt
- 1 ¼ tsp. kosher salt (or tsp. of regular salt)
- 4 ½ cups cooked brown rice

In a medium pot, combine the lentils, carrots, and enough water to cover by 1 inch. Simmer until the lentils are tender but not mushy, 12-20 minutes. Remove from the heat and drain. In a large saute pan, heat the oil over medium heat. Saute the onion until browned, about 10 minutes. Add the garlic and ginger and cook for 30 seconds. Stir in the tomatoes and half the apples and simmer for 10 minutes. Remove from the heat and stir in lentils and yogurt. Season with up to 1 ¼ tsp. kosher salt. Garnish wih the remaining apple. Serve with rice. Serves 6.2

Per Serving (1 cup lentils + ¾ cup rice) *Calories: 450 Sodium: 460 mg Total Fat: 12g Cholesterol: 10 mg Sat Fat: 1.5g Carbohydrates 71g Protein: 14g Fiber: 16g*

Taking Care of Your Incision

You will be given instructions regarding your dressing. As a rule, keep your incisions dry. You should avoid tub baths until your doctor says it is okay. Most abdominal incisions are closed with staples or absorbable sutures that dissolve and do not need to be removed in the postoperative period. The surgical incision may be held closed with Steri-Strips, which are thin pieces of paper tape that are placed across the incision and will easily peel off or fall off as the incision heals. The incision may be sealed with Dermabond or SurgiSeal, which are liquid skin adhesives that act like a superglue and allow you to get the incision wet without worry of infection. Depending on the size and location, incisions may also be closed with sutures or staples that are removed by the doctor or the nurse after the procedure, usually 7 to 10 days for sutures and 3 to 6 days for staples.

If you have had a vaginal operation, you also may have packing inside the vagina, which is removed one or two days after the surgery. This pack is placed in the vagina to prevent the accumulation of blood after surgery and does not cause any pain but does feel like pressure inside your vagina when it is removed slowly.

You can decrease the redness of your incision by putting vitamin A and/or vitamin E ointment on the incision. Ask your doctor if he/she approves of the use of these creams or ointments.

Feeling Better Emotionally

It is natural to feel a little depressed or blue following surgery. No one ever heals or returns to all activities as quickly as she would like. Although older women may experience less pain than younger women, they may take longer to recover than younger women. It is quite common to be easily fatigued after surgery. You may even find yourself wanting to take an afternoon nap; go ahead! This response to surgery is quite normal and will help your healing.

For big operations (such as abdominal surgery), six to eight weeks may be required before you have returned to your preoperative energy level. Just remember it takes time to recover from pelvic surgery. So go slowly. Your doctor will tell you when you can drive a car, return to work, and resume sexual intimacy.

It is also normal to lose muscle mass and strength after surgery, especially if recovery time is prolonged. If you are confined to the bed for several days or weeks, you can lose 1 to 5 percent of muscle mass per day. Older women tend to lose more than younger women, and this is a result of decreased growth hormone in older women, which is why it is important to begin moving around as soon as you can after the surgery. If you are in the hospital, the nurses will encourage you to sit up in bed, move into a chair, and exercise as much as and as soon as possible.

Nutritional deficiencies may also contribute to muscle loss, and that is another reason that a good diet is essential to healing and a prompt recovery. It is important to walk around at least three times a day. While you are in bed, you should flex your feet back and forth for several minutes a few times a day. This will help prevent blood clots from forming in the lower extremities. Having said that, currently, most surgeries are performed in a minimally invasive fashion, and you can expect to have less pain, a shorter recovery period, and to be back to your normal activities in much less time than in the past.

The website www.hystersisters.com is a great Internet resource for hysterectomy information, support, and recovery. HysterSisters contains credible information from women around the world who have faced hysterectomy firsthand. The site gives women tips and suggestions that are useful before hysterectomy, after hysterectomy, treatment options, surgical procedures, hormonal issues, emotional recovery, and a step-by-step guide through the weeks before and after surgery. We recommend this site to our patients and highly recommend it to our readers.

When to Call the Doctor

Most surgical procedures proceed without complications or problems in the postoperative period. However, there are certain conditions and situations when it is important to notify your physician.

If you develop fever, greater than 100°F, or chills, contact your doctor. This may be the result of a wound infection, a urinary tract infection, or pneumonia. The first sign of an infection is malaise and fever.

Check your incision every day. If there is increasing redness or a discharge from the incision, you should contact your physician as he/she may place you on antibiotics.

If you develop heavy bleeding from the vagina (i.e., one pad an hour), or if the bleeding from your vagina increases, then you need to call your doctor.

If you are unable to urinate or have prolonged constipation, there are a few things to consider. The simplest way to prevent constipation is to drink appropriate amounts of fluid daily (eight cups) and to take walks. Your doctor will also send you home with stool softeners, and some will also give you a prescription for laxatives when you are discharged from the hospital. These will often do the trick. If you do develop the inability to empty your bladder, then you will have to return to see your doctor.

The pain should begin to diminish after a few days. If the pain increases or if the pain is not relieved by pain medication, then you should call your doctor. If you have had an abdominal operation, and you experience distension of the abdomen, or any leakage from the site of your laparoscopy, you should contact your physician. Also, it is not normal to be nauseated or to have vomiting. If these occur, then you should go the emergency room.

The Bottom Line

Surgery is a stressful situation. The more you know about the surgery, including what happens before, during, and after the procedure, the easier it will be for you to go through the process and hasten your recovery. If you approach the surgery with a realistic expectation of what to expect before and after the procedure, your recovery will be very smooth and uneventful.

Chapter Thirteen

Managing Stress to Make Everything Feel Better Down There: A Guide for Wellness

It is an undeniable truth that stress can make many medical conditions worse. We do not know if stress causes the medical problems or if the medical problems are the contributors to the stress. This chapter will not take a position on causation. However, we will point out that many of the conditions we discuss in the book such as pelvic pain, menopause, interstitial cystitis, premenstrual syndrome, urinary and fecal incontinence, and female sexual dysfunction are certainly made worse when there is added stress in a woman's life. We hope to provide you with suggestions for reducing stress in your life and provide you with coping strategies if stress is impacting conditions in your pelvis.

The Stress Cycle

In order to understand the impact that stress has on our health, we need to go back thousands of years to when man lived in a cave and had to worry about the sabertoothed tiger that might enter the cave and hurt the caveman and his family. Primitive man developed a fight-or-flight response that prepared the caveman to fight the tiger or to flee and run from the cave to protect his family. When this primitive response is elicited in a modern woman or man who perceives a threat or danger, several events take place. With the perception of imminent danger, the nerve cells release chemicals like adrenaline, noradrenalin, and cortisol into the bloodstream.

The release of these chemicals triggers blood flow away from the digestive tract and the pelvis into the muscles of the arms and legs, which makes it possible to run away from the danger. Your heart and respiratory rates also increase, sending more oxygen to your legs in order to outrun the threat and get out of harm's way. Other changes include a dilation of the pupils, improved eyesight, increased awareness, and the ability to be clearly focused on removing yourself from danger. There is also an activation of your immune system, and even your ability to perceive pain is diminished; this allows you to get out of harm's way even if you are injured in some way.

This hard-wired stress response is your body's way of protecting you from danger. If the stress response is working properly, it helps you stay focused, energetic, and alert. In an emergency, this stress response can save your life, giving you increased physical strength to protect yourself and your loved ones.

When the fight or flight reaction is triggered, our body is flooded with cortisol and adrenaline, which makes us strong and ready to take on the danger of that sabertoothed tiger. It is this very reaction that allows soccer moms to pick up a car off a trapped child, something she wouldn't be able to accomplish under normal, non-stressed conditions. So the fight-or-flight response helps to preserve our species and protect us from outside dangers and stressors. When we face very real dangers to our physical survival, the fight-or-flight response is invaluable.

Unfortunately, our bodies cannot differentiate the sabertoothed tiger at the cave entrance from a missed deadline at the office. Additionally, our bodies and brains have not caught up with the twenty-first century. Today, our threat response is triggered by being late for carpool, waiting in the reception area in a doctor's office, having an argument with our spouses or our children, or hundreds of other outside events that make our bodies go into fight-or-flight mode, even though the danger to our physical well-being is very low. However, the reaction that occurs in our bodies is just the same: our brains trigger our bodies to increase cortisol and adrenaline into the bloodstream, our heart rates rise, and blood supply is redirected away from the stomach into the large muscles of the arms and legs.

When stress occurs multiple times a day and occurs day after day, the stress stops being helpful and starts causing deleterious changes to your health. It not only affects your bodily functions, but also your productivity, your relationship with others, and ultimately your quality of life.

In today's society, the nonstop stress means that your fight-or-flight alarm system never shuts off and is in the constant on position. Medical science has discovered that repeated stress, multiple times each day, leads to a build up of stress hormones. These hormones and chemicals, which are useful and necessary for short-term stresses, become harmful if present in large quantities or are not removed by body metabolism. As a result, these hormones that are repeatedly flooding the organs of the body for extended periods of time can lead to disorders like hypertension, headache, gastrointestinal disorders (Crohn's disease, ulcerative colitis, irritable bowel syndrome); can affect the immune system; render us more susceptible to infection, chronic fatigue, and depression. Although stress will exacerbate all of the conditions in the pelvis that we have written about in this book, it can have a major impact on pelvic pain, interstitial cystitis, incontinence, overactive bladder, and female sexual dysfunction.

Exactly how stress causes and contributes to disease is a question of particular interest to researchers. Women under stress sleep poorly and are less likely to exercise; they adopt poor eating habits, smoke more, and don't comply with medical treatment. Stress also triggers a response by the body's endocrine system, which releases hormones that affect the immune system and other biological systems in the body. Medical research has confirmed a direct link between real medical diseases and stress. There are estimates that 40 to 80 percent of all visits to doctors may be directly related to stress—that is, diseases either caused by stress or made worse by it.

Stress Relief to the Rescue

The first step in successful stress relief is the recognition that stress is partly or wholly responsible for many of your medical problems. The symptoms of excessive stress include a fast heartbeat, fast breathing, sweating and sweaty palms, back pain, a stiff neck and/or tight shoulders, and gastrointestinal complaints such as diarrhea, nausea, and abdominal pains. The next step is to identify those situations or events that trigger the stress in your life. Some stress triggers are blatantly obvious. Examples are recent divorce, personal or spousal job loss, caring for an elderly parent, and stresses associated with work or family. The daily hassles of carpool, waiting in the doctor's reception area, or deadlines associated with work can also contribute to your stress level. It is necessary to identify and to accept the responsibility for the stress triggers in your life. Only then will you be able to gain control of your stress and have the opportunity to reduce the symptoms in your pelvis.

Perhaps one of the best suggestions is to keep a stress journal. Just like keeping an incontinence journal, a stress journal will help you identify patterns of behavior that culminate in stress and the subsequent symptoms that can cause havoc and impact your quality of life.

A stress journal consists of first identifying what events are associated with stress. Then record how the stress impacted your symptoms. For example, if you are experiencing stress associated with deadlines at work, how did this affect your urinary symptoms or the pain in your pelvis? Then, if possible, find out what made you feel better. Was it exercise, a warm bath, or a hot fudge sundae? Certainly, the last is not going to be a problem solver and will only add to the guilt associated with the stressful circumstances.

A stress journal will help you keep track of what stress relievers work and which ones are ineffective. If keeping a written journal is cumbersome, you can use your smartphone to keep these helpful notes. If one stress reliever doesn't work, try another one. Now you won't have trouble remembering which stress relievers work and which are ineffective because you can easily go back and refer to your stress journal.

What *Not* to Do for Stress

Some options for coping with stress can make matters worse. Diving into a hot fudge sundae or eating chips or pizza is not going to help your stress level. Smoking and drinking too much alcohol (more than two drinks per day) is destructive.

By taking some time to develop more positive, health-enhancing options to relieve stress you not only will feel more balanced and less stressed, but also give your body a chance to strengthen in all ways.

The Four As of Dealing with Stress

1. **Avoid the stressor:** Try to limit your contact with people who drain your positive energy. If you know that being around Aunt Mary makes you anxious, especially when she asks you repeatedly why you aren't married, then make every effort to remove yourself from that situation. You don't have to attend every function where Aunt Mary will be present.

2. **Alter the stressor:** If you find that you are anxious and stressed out about carpools, then find ways to reduce the stress by making an effort to arrive 10 minutes early to pick up the kids and wait in line with a book to read, a tape to listen to, or a puzzle to do. All these options are acceptable and certainly reduce the stress that accompanies being in a rush to be on time in order to avoid having the children and the teachers upset that you are late.

3. **Adapt to the stressor:** If you can't control the stress, change yourself. You will find that you can adapt to stressful situations and regain your sense of control by changing your expectations and your attitude. For example, you can reframe the problem. If you are held up in traffic, you can use this opportunity to listen to a motivational tape, or use this down time to learn a new language. Another adaptation technique is to focus on the positive and all the good things that are happening to you. It has been shown that the human brain can't be attentive to both positive and negative thoughts at the same time. So you can reduce the negativity by focusing on the positive aspects of your life rather than the problems in the pelvis. Think about your blessings and banish your troubles, and you will find your stress will melt away.

4. **Accept the stressor:** When all else fails, give in to the stressor. If public speaking creates stress and it is unavoidable, then you just have to bite the bullet and accept this stressor if you want to continue speaking. If your teenage child's room is a mess and in disarray and this is a source of stress to you, you may just have to accept this situation and learn not to comment about the disarray in the room or have a confrontation with the child about the situation. It may be a whole lot easier to just close the door to the child's room. Try to follow the advice in Reinhold Niebuhr's serenity prayer: "Grant me the courage to change the things I can change, the serenity to accept the things I can't change, and the wisdom to know the difference."

Stress Relievers: Top 10-plus Picks to Tame Stress

Is stress making you angry, frustrated, and irritable? Stress relievers can help restore calm and serenity to your chaotic life. You don't have to invest a lot of time or thought into stress relievers. When your stress is getting out of control and you need quick stress relief, just try one of these stress relievers. According to the famed Mayo Clinic, there are effective stress relievers known to help people cope with difficult or challenging situations and feel better. We have also added a few other helpful suggestions.

Your Best Stress Reducers*

1. **Get active.** Virtually any form of exercise and physical activity can act as a stress reliever. Aerobic exercise, or increasing your heart rate, is the most effective, because it increases oxygen circulation and produces endorphins—chemicals that make you feel happy. To get the maximum benefit, aim for 150 minutes of aerobic exercise each week (or about 40 minutes, 4 times per week). Even if you're not an athlete or you're out of shape, exercise is still a good stress reliever. Physical activity pumps up your endorphins and refocuses your mind on your body's movements—improving your mood and helping the day's irritations fade away. Consider walking, jogging, gardening, house cleaning, biking, swimming, weightlifting, or anything else that gets you active.

2. **Good nutrition.** Part of having a healthy lifestyle is to have a healthy diet. A well-nourished and healthy person is better able to deal with stress than a person who is unhealthy and who consumes large quantities of alcohol, caffeine, and carbohydrate-loaded foods. Try to start out your day with a healthy breakfast and eat plenty of fresh fruits and vegetables and a diet that has 30 grams of fiber each day.

3. **Meditate.** During meditation, you focus your attention and eliminate the stream of jumbled thoughts that may be crowding your mind and causing stress. Meditation instills a sense of calm, peace, and balance that benefits both your emotional well-being and your overall health. Guided meditation, guided imagery, visualization, and other forms of meditation can be practiced anywhere at any time, whether you're out for a walk, riding the bus to work, or waiting at the doctor's office. This relaxation response can return your body to a healthy condition by reducing the stress hormones, slowing down your heart rate, reducing your blood pressure and relieving tension in your muscles.

4. **Laugh.** A good sense of humor can't cure all ailments, but it can help you feel better, even if you have to force a fake laugh through your grumpiness. When you start to laugh, it lightens your mental

load and actually causes positive physical changes in your body. Laughter fires up and then cools down your stress response and increases your heart rate and blood pressure, producing a good, relaxed feeling. Laughter also increases endorphins, which are more potent than morphine for pain relief. So read some jokes, tell some jokes, watch a comedy or hang out with your funny friends.

Several years ago, Norman Cousins, who was the editor of the *Saturday Evening Post*, had a severe debilitating condition, ankylosing spondylitis, and used humor to help himself recover and to control the pain so he no longer needed pain medications. He wrote about his experience, and *The Anatomy of An Illness As Seen By the Patient* was a best-selling book for several years and was mandatory reading for medical students throughout the country. This book is highly recommended for those suffering from chronic medical problems especially those associated with disorders in the pelvis.

5. **Connect.** When you're stressed and irritable, your instinct may be to wrap yourself in a cocoon. Instead, reach out to family and friends and make social connections. Social contact is a good stress reliever because it can distract you, provide support, help you weather life's up and downs, and make you feel good by doing good. So take a coffee break with a friend, e-mail a relative, volunteer for a charitable group, or visit your place of worship. Friends are helpful and empathetic. They may not be able to solve your problem, but they can help you get the stress off your chest and out into the open. A close friend who can be trusted with your feelings and your discomfort is an invaluable resource.

6. **Assert yourself.** You might want to do it all, but you probably can't, at least not without paying a price. Learn to say no to some tasks or to delegate them. Saying yes may seem like an easy way to keep the peace, prevent conflicts, and get the job done right. But it may actually cause you internal conflict because your needs and those of your family come second, which can lead to stress, anger, resentment, and even the desire to exact revenge. And that's not very calm and peaceful. When you are asked to be on a committee or attend a function that isn't in your best interest, learn to say no gracefully, and explain that accepting that obligation would add stress to your life and you already have enough of that. Good friends and those that ask for your time and energy will certainly understand.

7. **Do yoga.** With its series of postures and controlled-breathing exercises, yoga is a popular stress reliever. Yoga brings together physical and mental disciplines to achieve peacefulness of body and mind, helping you relax and manage stress and anxiety. Try yoga on your own or find a class—you can find classes in most communities. Hatha yoga, in particular, is a good stress reliever because of its slower pace and easier movements.

8. **Sleep.** Stress often gives sleep the heave-ho. You have too much to do—and too much to think about—and your sleep suffers. But sleep is the time when your brain and body recharge. And the quality and amount of sleep you get affects your mood, energy level, concentration, and overall functioning. If you have sleep troubles, make sure that you have a quiet, relaxing bedtime routine, listen to soothing music, put clocks away, avoid caffeine and alcohol especially in the evening before going to bed, and stick to a consistent schedule—go to sleep at the same time each evening and wake up at the same time each morning. Another important part of achieving good sleep hygiene is to dedicate the bedroom for sleep and sex only and do work elsewhere.

9. **Journal.** Writing out thoughts and feelings can be a good release for otherwise pent-up emotions. Don't think about what to write—just let it happen. Write whatever comes to mind. No one else needs to read it, so don't strive for perfection in grammar or spelling. Just let your thoughts flow on paper—or computer screen. Once you're done, you can toss out what you wrote or save it to reflect on later. Who knows, you just may be able to convert that journal into a book and be on the *New York Times* best-seller list!

10. **Get musical.** Listening to or playing music is a good stress reliever because it provides a mental distraction, reduces muscle tension, and decreases stress hormones. Crank up the volume and let your mind be absorbed by the music. If music isn't your thing, though, turn your attention to another hobby you enjoy, such as gardening, sewing, sketching—anything that requires you to focus on what you're doing rather than on your pain or your stress. Today there are so many options in addition to music that can be relaxing and can reduce stress, such as meditation, books on tape, and listening to or watching podcasts.

11. **Seek counsel.** If new stressors are challenging your ability to cope or if self-care stress relievers just aren't relieving your stress, you may

need to look for reinforcements in the form of professional therapy or counseling. Therapy may be a good idea if stress leaves you feeling overwhelmed or trapped, if you worry excessively, or if you have trouble carrying out daily routines or meeting responsibilities at work, home, or school. Professional counselors or therapists can help you identify sources of your stress and teach you new coping tools.

12. **Get a massage**. Stress leads to contraction of your muscles and the build up of lactic acid. A good massage relaxes the muscles and dissipates the toxic lactic acid. If you don't want to have a massage, a warm bath or a few minutes in the hot tub can also do wonders. There are also many self-massage techniques that you can employ to relax and reduce stress. For example, you can place your thumbs behind your ears while spreading your fingers on to the side of your head. By moving your fingers back and forth slightly in a circular fashion with your fingertips for 15 to 30 seconds, you can achieve a sense or relaxation and stress relief.

13. **Now there's an app for that.** Did you know that there is an online application for stress reduction? Stress Reducer is a free app, which shows photos of seashells. By touching the seashell on the app, you can hold the iPhone to your ear and you can hear the ocean waves through the shell. You close your eyes, take a deep breath, and relax. Each shell has a different sound from waves crashing to seagulls and other ocean or sea sounds. The only thing missing is the smell of the ocean!

    Another app, Stress Tracker, is a personal stress management app that tracks, identifies, and helps relieve your daily stress. A team of clinical psychologists and researchers developed the program. The program counteracts and balances the effects of stress as well as helps you gain clarity in difficult and stressful situations.

14. **Meditation and Prayer.** Many people turn to their spiritual communities or religions for emotional support and comfort. Attending religious services, praying at home, or performing religious rituals is known to help many relieve stress

*Adapted with permission from Mayo Clinic.

The Bottom Line

Stress is an integral part of many of the problems located in a woman's pelvis. Stress reduction is part and parcel of the treatment for many of these conditions. However, one size does not fit all. No single method will work for all women who suffer or are impacted with problems in the pelvis. Stress may not be able to be entirely eliminated. But the good news is that stress can be controlled. Find out what works for you and get a handle on your stress and reduce your symptoms and your discomfort.

A Final Note

All women older than 40 years of age have issues and challenges with some aspect of their pelvic tissues or down there. You should not suffer in silence.

We have written this book because many women are uncomfortable discussing these issues with their friends, their partners, and even with their doctors. The truth is that the organs of your pelvis can be the most celebrated area of your body—and they should be.

This book represents a compilation of stories from women just like you—women who have experienced similar challenges and uncertainties down there.

We want you to recognize that help is available. Your road to recovery begins with understanding your problem and the underlying symptoms, pain, or discomfort you are experiencing. The next step is to speak to your doctor who will then craft a plan of action or refer you to the type of doctor who can help you with *all* of your problems *down there*. Finally, you must take responsibility for executing your personal plan of action. Remember, to know and not to do is just the same as not to know. Be a partner with your doctor and follow the course of action that is laid out for you. Only then will you gain control of the issues with your tissues.

This book should serve as guide to help make you a better patient. Hopefully, you will read this book before your appointment with your doctor. Now, you are in a position to understand your doctor's advice—and you have the knowledge necessary to help your doctor reach an accurate diagnosis and start you on the road to recovery.

We also want to empower you to develop a support system with which you can discuss what is going on down there—whether it's your physician, your support group, your partner, your friends, your relatives, or your book club (discussed on the next page)—it's important to feel comfortable and confident sharing your troubles and triumphs, seeking advice from those who have been down this road before and sharing your experiences with those who are still striving to understand what is going on down there.

Finally, we would like to hear from you. If you have a success story, please share it with us so we can help others learn from your experience. Also, if you are grappling with a challenge, perhaps we can connect you to someone who can help. You can reach us at www.WomensHealthDownThere.com.

The *Down There* Book Club

What do you picture when you think of a book club? We envision a group of people sitting around a room, sipping tea, reading verses from a poem, or debating the meaning of a metaphor. Discussing nonfiction books at a book club can be fun and educational. In fact, many nonfiction picks of Oprah's Book Club have demonstrated that nonfiction books can be a wonderful way to open up your eyes to new information and experiences. We want to encourage and support forming *Down There* book clubs in your area so that you can share and discuss what you've learned with others and listen to their unique perspectives. When you start talking about the issues with your pelvic tissues, not only will it help you to connect with others, including family, who are having similar experiences, but you also will be able to communicate better with your doctor.

You can come up with discussion topics for your own book club. Have each member write down one open-ended question before the meeting. You can find more suggestions at www.book-clubs-resource.com. The following are some book club discussion suggestions for *What's Going on Down There?*:

- ♦ What was unique about *What's Going on Down There?* and how did it enhance your understanding of your pelvic area?
- ♦ What themes did the authors emphasize in *What's Going on Down There*?
- ♦ What is the message that the authors are trying to get across to the reader?
- ♦ How has reading *What's Going on Down There?* changed your opinion of women's pelvic health?
- ♦ What was one thing you learned from *What's Going on Down There?* that you did not know was possible?

- Did certain parts of *What's Going on Down There?* make you uncomfortable? If so, why did you feel that way? Did this lead to a new understanding of yourself?
- Why do you believe so many women suffer in silence from these down-there conditions?
- Did *What's Going on Down There?* change your life in a positive or negative way? Explain
- Will you read any future books by these authors?
- How do you feel this book will help you communicate better with your doctor?
- Do you or anyone you know experience the symptoms manifested by any of the women in the stories from the various chapters? How are your symptoms similar or different than those described in the stories?
- How has *What's Going on Down There?* increased your interest in women's health issues?

If you're starting your own book club, the following information may help you. Here are the most popular tidbits regarding book clubs:

- Where are good places to hold book club meetings?
  Home; restaurant; library; community center; meeting rooms at your gym; café with private rooms; rent a movie theater, discuss book, then watch a movie; hotel lobby; or room
- Where do you recruit people for your book club?
  Friends, coworkers, post flyers at library or local café
- How many people make a good-sized book club?
  Six to 10
- How often should you have these book club meetings?
  Usually once a month
- How do you decide on the process of choosing books to discuss in your book club?
  Usually members can write down names of one to three books, and then everyone can vote on their favorites.

- What should you serve during a traditional book club when discussing *What's going on Down There?* (taken from *Down There Diet* list)
    - Decaf tea
    - Nonwheat crackers
    - Non-aged cheese
    - Fresh fruit
    - Fresh, raw veggies

What Do These Words Mean on My Surgical Consent?
Glossary of *Down There* Operations

Surgical Procedure	Also Known As/Common Examples	English Please!	Chapter?
Sling	• Suburethral sling • Midurethral sling • TVT • TOT • Mini-sling • Single-incision sling • Fascia sling • Synthetic sling	A material (usually polypropylene) that looks like tape and is a quarter of an inch wide is placed underneath the urethra to support it; slings have a very high success rate for stress urinary incontinence.	Two
Burch	• Burch colposuspension • Burch retropubic urethropexy • Retropubic operation	This surgical technique uses sutures to suspend the vagina to Cooper's ligament. This procedure can be performed via abdominal, laparoscopic, or robotic routes; Burch has high success rate for stress urinary incontinence.	Two

Bulking agent injection	• Periurethral bulking agent injection • Urethral injection • Coaptite • Durasphere • Macroplastique • Solesta	Like collagen injection in your lips, the inside of the urethra is "plumped-up" using different materials (Macroplastique, Coaptite, or Durasphere); can be helpful for stress urinary incontinence; Solesta is helpful for fecal incontinence.	Two, Seven
Neuromodulation	• Sacral neuromodulation • InterStim • Neurostimulation • Bladder or bowel pacemaker	An thin wire is inserted next to the sacral nerves (below the spinal cord); stimulation of these nerves by a pacemaker is effective for severe overactive bladder syndrome and also for bowel control disorder.	Two, Seven
Posterior tibial nerve stimulation	• PTNS	Similar to acupuncture, a small needle is placed in the ankle and stimulated in order to improve overactive bladder symptoms.	Two
Intravesical botulinum toxin injection	• Bladder Botox injection • Intravesical injection	In this procedure, 100 to 200 units of Botox are injected inside the back wall of the bladder in order to improve severe overactive bladder symptoms.	Two

Laparoscopic surgery	• Laparoscopy • Laparoscopic sacral colpopexy (L-SCP)	This is a type of minimally invasive surgery where small keyhole incisions are made in the belly; rigid instruments and a small camera are inserted through the keyholes in order to perform a given operation.	Three
Robotic surgery	• Davinci surgery • Robotic-assisted laparoscopic surgery • Robotic-assisted laparoscopic hysterectomy (R-TLH) • Robotic-assisted laparoscopic sacral colpopexy (R-SCP)	This is a type of minimally invasive surgery where small keyhole incisions are made in the belly, flexible instruments attached to robotic arms are inserted through the keyholes, and the operation is performed by a surgeon who controls sophisticated joysticks.	Three
Vaginal surgery	• High uterosacral ligament colposuspension (HUSLS) • Sacrospinous ligament fixation (SSLF) • Anterior colporrhaphy (a.k.a. anterior repair, "AR," cystocele repair) • Posterior colporrhaphy (a.k.a. posterior repair, "PR," rectocele repair)	This is a type of minimally invasive surgery where no incisions are made in the belly and all of the operation is performed through the natural orifice, the vagina. Various procedures can be performed by this technique using sutures only.	Three

Anterior repair	• Anterior colporrhaphy • Cystocele repair	This procedure repairs the stretch and tear of the pubocervical septum, thus re-establishing the separation between the bladder and the vagina. The bladder sits on top of the pubocervical septum, which is like a hammock of support.	Three
Posterior repair	• Posterior colporrhaphy • Posterior colpo-perineorrhaphy • Rectocele repair	This procedure repairs the stretch and tear of the rectovaginal septum, thus re-establishing the separation between the walls of the rectum and vagina.	Three
Perineorrhaphy	• Colpo-perineorrhaphy	This procedure reduces the opening of the vagina and adds distance between the anus and vagina.	Three
Vaginal mesh for prolapse	• Mesh kits • Vaginal mesh kits	This is a type of vaginal surgery used to repair pelvic organ prolapse, where a pre-shaped sheet of synthetic mesh is inserted through the vagina. These procedures are now under investigation (522 trials) to determine whether they are safe and effective.	Three

Sacral colpopexy (SCP)	• Sacrocolpopexy • Colposacropexy • Laparoscopic sacral colpopexy (L-SCP) • Robotic-assisted laparoscopic sacral colpopexy (R-SCP)	This is an operation that repairs pelvic organ prolapse. A piece of Y-shaped polypropylene is attached to the back (rectovaginal septum and front (pubocervical septum) of the vagina and then attached to a ligament over the sacrum. The operation can be performed by abdominal (A-SCP) incision or by laparoscopic (L-SCP) or robotic (R-SCP) technique.	Three
Sacrohysteropexy	• Uterus preserving procedure for POP • Sacrocolpo-cervico-hysteropexy	This surgical technique, which is a variation of a sacral colpopexy, is used to repair pelvic organ prolapse without performing a hysterectomy. During this procedure, the vagina, cervix, and lower uterus are suspended to the ligament over the sacrum using polypropylene mesh and sutures.	Three

Sacral-colpocervicopexy (SCCP)	• Repairing POP after a partial hysterectomy	This surgical technique, which is a variation of sacral colpopexy, is used to repair pelvic organ prolapse without performing a total hysterectomy. During this procedure, the vagina and cervix are suspended to the sacrum with polyproylene mesh; this procedure usually is performed immediately after a partial hysterectomy.	Three
Colpectomy	• Vaginectomy • Total colpectomy • Partial colpectomy	This is a vaginal procedure where the skin of the vagina is removed.	Three
Colpocleisis	• LeForte procedure • LeForte colpocleisis	This is a vaginal procedure for prolapse where the vagina is closed.	Three
Radiofrequency Procedure	• Renessa (for urethra) • Secca (for anal canal)	Radiofrequency energy is used to heat tissue (either urethra or anal canal) so that the tissue can shrink and tighten; can be helpful for stress urinary incontinence and fecal incontinence.	Two, Seven

Enterocystoplasty	• Bladder augmentation	Surgery which enlarges the bladder by attaching a piece of intestine to it.	Four
Ileal conduit	• Bricker ileal conduit • Urostomy	This procedure is done for patients whose bladder is removed. The ureters are redirected from the bladder into a piece of small intestine that has been shaped into a pouch which is then attached to the abdominal wall. Urine goes from the kidneys, down the ureters, to the pouch, and then out through the belly into an ostomy bag, which must be emptied periodically.	Four
Pudendal nerve decompression	• Pudendal neuralgia surgery	This is a surgical procedure for patients with pudendal nerve pain where an incision is made over the buttocks, the muscles are separated, the ligaments are cut, the pudendal nerve is released, scar tissue is reduced, and ligaments are re-attached.	Five

			Seven
Rectovaginal fistula repair	• Transvaginal rectovaginal fistula repair • Transperineal rectovaginal fistula repair • Transanal rectovaginal fistula repair (anorectal advancement) • Perineo-proctotomy	This procedure is used to close an abnormal communication between the vagina and rectum.	
Total abdominal hysterectomy (TAH)	• Total hysterectomy • Abdominal hysterectomy	In this surgery, the uterus and the cervix are removed by making a bikini incision on your belly. The ovaries and fallopian tubes are not removed by TAH.	Ten
Supracervical hysterectomy (SCH)	• Partial hysterectomy	In this surgery, the uterus is removed but the cervix is not removed; the ovaries and fallopian tubes are not removed. It may be done through the abdomen or by laparoscopic or robotic techniques.	Ten

Vaginal hysterectomy (TVH)	• Transvaginal hysterectomy • Total vaginal hysterectomy	In this surgery, the uterus and cervix are removed through the vagina (no cuts on your belly). The ovaries and fallopian tubes are not removed by TVH.	Ten
Total laparoscopic hysterectomy (TLH)	• TLH	In this surgery, the uterus and the cervix are removed; the operation is done through small keyhole incisions. The ovaries and fallopian tubes are not removed by TLH. This surgery can also be performed using Robotic technology.	Ten
Laparoscopically assisted vaginal hysterectomy (LAVH)	• LAVH	This is a mixture of TVH and TLH. In this surgery, the uterus and the cervix are removed; part of the operation is done through keyhole incisions on your belly and part is done through an incision in the vagina. The uterus is removed through the vagina. The ovaries and fallopian tubes are not removed by LAVH.	Ten

Bilateral salpingo-oophorectomy (BSO)	• Removal of gonads • Removal of ovaries	In this surgery, both ovaries and fallopian tubes are removed. The term "BSO" can be added to any of the hysterectomy procedures described above; BSO can be done by abdominal, laparoscopic, or robotic techniques.	Ten
D and C	• Dilatation and curettage • D & C • Hysteroscopy with D & C • Fractional D & C	The cervix is opened and the inside of the uterus is first visualized with a camera (hysteroscopy); then the inside lining of the uterus is shaved.	Ten
Uterine artery embolization (UAE)		A catheter is threaded into the femoral vein, in the thigh, and particles are injected into the uterine arteries in order to block them.	Ten
Myomectomy	• Uterus preserving procedure for fibroids	One or few fibroids are removed from the uterus without removing the uterus itself. This is usually done by laparoscopic or robotic technique.	Ten

Endometrial ablation (EMB)	• Novasure (radiofrequency) • Hydro ThermaAblator (water) • Cryoablation (freezing) • ThermaChoice (balloon) • Microsulis (microwave)	The lining of the uterus is either heated to a high temperature or cooled to a low temperature in order to destroy the inside lining; this procedure preserves the uterus.	Ten
Progestin IUD	• Mirena • Levonorgestrel IUD	A quarter-sized, T-shaped piece of plastic that contains the progestogen called levonorgestrel is inserted into the uterus.	Ten
Radical trachalectomy		This procedure can be an alternative to a hysterectomy for those with early cervical cancer who desire to have children. During this procedure, only the cervix and the surrounding tissues are removed, but the uterus is left intact.	Ten

Vaginal rejuvenation	• Vaginoplasty • Posterior colpo-perineorrhaphy (for non-medical reasons) • Perineorrhaphy	The vaginal opening is reduced in size; can be done with scalpel, laser, or other high-energy device.	Eleven
Labiaplasty	• Labial reduction • Labia minora excision • Labial contouring • Barbie	The small lips (labia minora) are reduced for either medical (labial hypertrophy) or cosmetic reasons.	Eleven
Labial injection	• Labia majora injection • Labial augmentation	This is an injection of fat into the labia minora to take away looseness and wrinkles and to make them appear smoother and fuller.	Eleven
G-spot amplification	• G-shot	This is an injection of a filler (e.g., Collagen) into the G-spot in an attempt to increase sexual pleasure during intercourse.	Eleven
Anal bleaching	• Anal lightening • Anal toning	Chemical is applied to the area around the anus in order to lighten the skin color.	Eleven

Hymenoplasty	• Hymen restoration • Re-virginization	The hymen is sutured and reconnected so as to re-establish continuity around the opening of the vagina.	Eleven
Clitoral unhooding	• Hoodectomy	This is removal of excess tissue around the clitoral hood or the removal of the clitoral hood either for hygienic, cosmetic, or sexual purpose.	Eleven

References

Abrams P, Andersson KE, Birder L, et al. Fourth International Consultation on Incontinence Recommendations of the International Scientific Committee: Evaluation and Treatment of Urinary Incontinence, Pelvic Organ Prolapse, and Fecal Incontinence. Neurourology and Urodynamics 29:213-240

ACOG Practice Bulletin No. 81. American College of Obstetricians and Gynecologists. Obstetrics and Gynecology 2007; 109:1233-48

Anderson GL, Limacher M, Assaf AR, et al. Effects of conjugated equine estrogen in postmenopausal women with hysterectomy: the Women's Health Initiative randomized controlled trial. Journal of the American Medical Association 2004; 291: 1701-12

Bachman G, Lobo R, Gut R, et al. Efficacy of Low-Dose Estradiol vaginal tablets in the treatment of atrophic vaginitis: a randomized controlled trial. Obstetrics and Gynecology 2008; 111(1): 67-76

Banu NS, Manyonda IT. Alternative medical and surgical options to hysterectomy. Best Practices and Research Clinical Obstetrics and Gynaecology 2005; 19(3): 431-49

Basson R, Berman J, Burnett A, et al. Report of the international consensus development conference on female sexual dysfunction: definitions and classifications. Journal of Urology 2000; 163:888-93

Basson R. Sexuality and sexual disorders. Clinical Update Women's Health Care 2003: II:1-94

Benjamin-Pratt AT, Howard FM. Management of chronic pelvic pain. Minerva Ginecol 2010; 62(5): 447-65

Cauley JA, Robbins J, Chen Z, et al. Effects of estrogen plus progestin on risk of fractures and bone mineral density: the Women's Health Initiative randomized trial. Journal of the American Medical Association 2003; 290: 1729-38

Chlebowski RT, Hendrix SL, Langer RD, et al. Influence of estrogen plus progestin on breast cancer and mammography in healthy postmenopausal women: the Women's Health Initiative randomized trial. Journal of the American Medical Association 2003; 289: 3243-53

Chronic pelvic pain. ACOG Practice Bulletin No. 51. American College of Obstetricians and Gynecologists. Obstetrics and Gynecology 2004; 103:589-605

Cohen LS, Miner C, Brown EW, et al. Premenstrual daily fluoxetine for premenstrual dysphoric disorder: a placebo-controlled, clinical trial using computerized diaries. Obstetrics and Gynecology 2002; 100: 435-44

Col NF, Hirota LK, Orr RK, et al. Hormone replacement therapy after breast cancer: a systematic review and quantitative assessment of risk. Journal of Clinical Oncology 2001: 19(8): 2357-63

Cushman M, Kuller LH, Prentice R, et al. Estrogen plus progestin and risk of venous thrombosis. Journal of the American Medical Association 2004; 292: 1573-80

Ettinger B, Grady D, Tosteson A. et al. Effects of the Women's Health Initiative on Women's Decisions to Discontinue Postmenopausal Hormone Therapy. Obstetrics and Gynecology 2003; 102(6): 1225-32

FitzGerald MP, Richter HE, Siddique S, et al. Colpocleisis: a review. Pelvic floor disorders network. International Urogynecology Journal Pelvic Floor Dysfunction 2006; 17:261-71

Grady-Weliky TA. Premenstrual dysphoric disorder. New England Journal of Medicine 2003; 348: 433-38

Graziottin A, Brotto LA. Vulvar vestibulitis syndrome: a clinical approach. Journal of Sex and Marital Therapy 2004; 30(3)

Hammoud A, Gago LA, Diamond MP. Adhesions in patients with chronic pelvic pain: a role for adhesiolysis? Fertility and Sterility 2004; 82(6):1483-91

College of Obstetricians and Gynecologists. Obstet Gynecol 2004; 104 (suppl)

Hibner M, Desai N, Robertson LJ, etal. Pudendal neuralgia. Journal of Minimally Invasive Gynecology 2010; 17(2): 148-153

Holmberg L, Iversen O, Magnus C, et al. Increased risk of recurrence after hormone replacement therapy in breast cancer survivors. Journal of the National Cancer Institute 100(7); 475-482

Karcaaltincaba M, Karcaaltinacaba D, Dogra VS. Pelvic congestion syndrome. Ultrasound Clinics 2008; 3(3): 415-425

Lethaby A, Hickey M, Garry R. Endometrial destruction techniques for heavy menstrual bleeding. The Cochrane Library 2009; DOI: 10.1002/14651858.CD001501.pub2

Longinotte MK, Jacobson GF, Hung Y, et al. Probability of hysterectomy after endometrial ablation. Obstetrics and Gynecology 2008; 112(6): 1214-1220

Magtibay P, Magrina J. Ovarian remnant syndrome. Clinical Obstetrics and Gynecology 2006; 49(3): 526-34

Magtibay PM, NYholm JL, Hernandez, et al. Ovarian remnant syndrome. American Journal of Obstetrics and Gynecology 2005; 193: 2062-66

Marjoribanks J, Lethaby A, Farquhar C. Surgery versus medical therapy for heavy menstrual bleeding. Cochrane Database of Systematic Reviews 2006, Issue 2. Art. No.: CD003855

Marshburn PB, Matthews ML, Hurst BS. Uterine artery embolization as a treatment option for uterine myomas. Obstetrics and Gynecology Clinics of North America 2006; 33:125-44

Newton K, Buist D, Keenan N. et al. Use of alternative therapies for menopausal symptoms: results of a population-based survey. Obstetrics and Gynecology 2002; 100(1): 18-25

Nygaard I, McCreery R, Brubaker L. Abdominal sacrocolpopexy: a comprehensive review. Obstetrics and Gynecology 2004; 104(4): 805-23

Osmundsen BC, Clark A, Goldsmity C, etal. Mesh erosion robotic sacrocolpopexy. Female Pelvic Medicine and Reconstructive Surgery 2012; 18(2): 86-88

Parker WH, Broder MS, Liu Z, et al. Ovarian conservation at the time of hysterectomy for benign disease. Obstetrics and Gynecology 2005; 106(2): 219-226

Prevalance, incidence and stability of premenstrual dysphoric disorder in the community. Psychological Medicine 2002; 32:119-132

Reed BD, Caron AM, Gorenflo DW, et al. Treatment of vulvodynia with tricyclic antidepressants: efficacy and associated factors. Journal of Lower Genital Tract Disease 2006: 10: 245-51

Rioux JE, Devlin C, Gelfand MM, et al. 17beta-estradiol vaginal tablet versus conjugated equine estrogen vaginal cream to relieve menopausal atrophic vaginitis. Menopause 2000; 7: 156-61

Rossouw JE, Anderson GL, Prentice RL, et al. Risks and benefits of estrogen plus progestin in healthy postmenopausal women: principal results from the Women's Health Initiative randomized controlled trial. Women's Health Initiative Steering Committee. Journal of the American Medical Association 2002; 288: 321-33

Saini J, Kuczynski E, Gretz HG, et al. Supracervical hysterectomy versus total abdominal hysterectomy: perceived effects on sexual function. BMC Womens Health 2002; 2(1)

Thakar R, Ayers S, Clarkson P, et al. Outcomes after total versus subtotal abdominal hysterectomy. New England Journal of Medicine 2002; 347: 1318-25

Wassertheil-Smoller S, Hendrix SL, Limacher M, et al. Effect of estrogen plus progestin on stroke in postmenopausal women: the Women's Health Initiative: a randomized trial. Journal of the American Medical Association 2003; 289: 2673-84

Weisberg E, Ayton E, Darling G, et al. Endometrial and vaginal effects of low-dose estradiol delivered by vaginal ring or vaginal tablet 2005; 8(1): 83-93

Welk BK, Teichman JM. Dyspareunia response in patients with interstitial cystitis treated with intravesical lidocaine, bicarbonate, and heparin. Urology 71(1): 67-70

Whitehead WE, Wald A, Norton NY. Treatment options for fecal incontinence. Dis Colon Rectum 2001; 44:131-42

Zullo MA, Plotti F, Calcagno M, et al. One-year follow-up of tension-free vaginal tape (TVT) and trans-obturator suburethral tape inside to outside (TVT-O) for surgical treatment of female stress urinary incontinence: a prospective randomized trial. European Urology 2007; 51(5): 1376-84

INDEX